Clinical Decision Making for Improving Prognosis

Rong Liu
Editor

Clinical Decision Making for Improving Prognosis

Science Press
Beijing

Springer

Editor
Rong Liu
Hepatopancreatobiliary Surgery
Chinese PLA General Hospital
Beijing, China

ISBN 978-981-19-2954-0 ISBN 978-981-19-2952-6 (eBook)
https://doi.org/10.1007/978-981-19-2952-6
Jointly published with Science Press
The print edition is not for sale in China (Mainland). Customers from China (Mainland) please order the print book from: Science Press.

This Springer imprint is published by the registered company Springer Nature Singapore Pte Ltd.
The registered company address is: 152 Beach Road, #21-01/04 Gateway East, Singapore 189721, Singapore

Abstract: Rapid advances of big data and artificial intelligence (AI) techniques have pushed the envelope of traditional surgery to intelligent surgery, which revolutionizes the traditional medicine model dominated by the experiences of interveners and evidence-based medicine. Intelligent surgery requires to judiciously integrate the clinical experience of interveners and medical evidence with the new AI techniques, so as to achieve the best therapeutic effect for patients through effective disease risk control. This book puts forward a new theory of prognostic control surgery in the long-term clinical practice of hepato-pancreato-biliary surgery. Our theory takes the optimal prognosis of patients as the goal, and pre-controls the disease risk through the best combination of the optimal intervener, intervention methods, and intervention timing to achieve the maximum clinical benefits for patients with minimal medical trauma. This theory also takes full advantage of information technologies such as neural networks, deep learning, big data, and imaging system and uses high-dimensional decision-making to replace the traditional two-dimensional decision-making tree model.

A main technical challenge in the theory is how to effectively exploit the AI techniques to improve the work efficiency of large hospitals, enhance the service level of primary medical care, and improve the diagnosis, prediction, and treatment of diseases. Prognostic control surgery advocates the exploitation of emerging information technology methods, such as medical image recognition and prediction, 3D reconstruction-based surgical planning, intraoperative navigation, and remote intelligent robotic surgical system, to promote the rapid and balanced surgical diagnosis and treatment.

Guided by our theory of prognosis control surgery, our team successfully established minimally invasive anatomic hepatectomy, individualized pancreatic surgical approaches, modular hepatectomy, single-layer continuous suture of pancreaticojejunostomy, and end-to-end pancreatic anastomosis. This book also provides details of four core surgical strategies proposed in our prognosis control surgery, namely, blood control technique, surgical approach selection, resection technique, and reconstruction technique, by which to achieve minimally invasive surgery regularization and complex surgery simplification.

Foreword

Recently, we have lived in a dramatically changing world. In our surgical field, there have been many innovations including robotic surgery, image-guided surgery, and high information technologies such as artificial intelligence (AI).

Just a few years ago, there were no legions of deep learning scientists developing intelligent products and services at major companies and startups. Recently, deep learning has taken the world by surprise, driving rapid progress in fields as diverse as computer vision, natural language processing, automatic speech recognition, reinforcement learning, and statistical modeling. With these advances in hand, we can now build cars that drive themselves, smart reply systems, wearable medical appliances, and so on. However, surgeons usually had no idea how machine learning could be helpful in surgery.

Professor Rong Liu's group proposes prognostic control surgery based on long-term and tremendous experiences on hepato-pancreato-biliary surgery.

They recommend that pre-controls the disease risk through the best combination of the optimal intervener, intervention methods, and timing to achieve the maximum clinical benefits from surgical stress. Those theories take full advantage of information technologies such as neural networks, deep learning, big data, and imaging system to replace traditional decision-making.

This book is designed to achieve minimally invasive surgery regularization and complex surgery simplification through prognosis control as well as standardization of surgical techniques. I hope this textbook would be loved by many surgeons to broaden their knowledge and safety on HBP surgery.

Department of Surgery
Seoul National University Hospital
Seoul, Korea

Jin-Young Jang

27 April 2019

Foreword

With the gradual application of information technology represented by the Internet, big data, and artificial intelligence, surgery has entered the era of intelligent surgery, and 3D reconstruction, intraoperative navigation, and robotic surgery have promoted the development of minimally invasive surgery. How to change the traditional diagnosis and treatment concept of doctors, how to make full use of advanced intelligent surgical tools, and how to better serve patients are the urgent issues that need to be solved at present.

As a pioneer of minimally invasive hepatobiliary and pancreatic surgery in China and abroad, Professor Rong Liu is not only a world leader in the number of robotic hepatobiliary and pancreatic surgeries but also has unique insights and innovations in surgical techniques and concepts. What is even more valuable is that Professor Rong Liu is not satisfied with his profound attainments in the field of surgery, but from the perspective of adapting to the rapid development of medical technology and the increasing medical needs of patients, he has proposed the theory of prognostic control surgery in his long-term surgical clinical practice.

Starting from the theory of prognosis control, "Prognosis Control Surgery" divides the surgical process into four major elements: disease risk, interventionist, intervention means, and intervention timing and elaborates them respectively. On this basis, four core strategies of surgery are summarized: blood control, access, resection, and reconstruction, emphasizing the maximum benefit to patients with minimal damage. This work is highly innovative and practical, overcoming the limitations of the traditional surgical medical model, and has important reference and learning value especially in the current rapid interactive development of information technology and surgery.

Wan Yee Lau

Chinese Academy of Sciences
Beijing, China

Lee Woo Sing College
The Chinese University of Hong Kong
Shatin, Hong Kong

16 April 2019

Foreword

Surgery has evolved significantly over the last few centuries changing from seemingly barbaric procedures to highly specialized procedures. There is an exponential growth in the number of complex operations being performed worldwide on a day-to-day basis. One of the main reasons for success is the ever-expanding availability of newer technologies. Having said this, we should admit the fact that we are still far from perfection, and there is scope for further refining the management strategies to achieve optimum results in our patients.

The powerful evolving technologies like artificial intelligence (AI), big data, and three-dimensional (3D) printing techniques are likely to have a significant impact on the future of medicine. The concept of "Prognosis Control Surgery" by Prof. Rong Liu is new and exciting, where the strategy would be to exploit artificial intelligence at every step of patient care from risk elimination to palliation. It has the potential to revolutionize the field of surgery just the way ether anesthesia revolutionized this field in the last century.

This book mainly focuses on the management of hepato-pancreato-biliary disorders, utilizing technologies like neural networks, deep learning, big data, and imaging system. Authors will also exploit methods as medical image recognition and prediction, a 3D reconstruction-based surgical planning, intraoperative navigation, and remote intelligent robotic surgical system to promote the rapid and balanced surgical diagnosis and treatment. This book is based on four core operational strategies, namely, blood control technique, surgical approach selection, resection technique, and reconstruction technique, by which to achieve minimally invasive surgery regularization and complex surgery simplification.

I hope this book by Prof. Rong Liu will help to advance the surgical sciences towards more customized and safe healthcare.

Best Wishes,

C. Palanivelu

Gastrointestinal Surgery
GEM Hospital & Research Centre
Coimbatore, Tamil Nadu, India
21 May 2019

Content Introduction

This book is divided into six chapters; the first chapter is Introduction: a total of five sections. Section 1 proposes the basic concept of prognosis control surgery and four elements of prognosis control surgery, and analyzes the ultimate goal, realization means, and realization process of prognosis control surgery. Sections 2 to 5 are summarized in terms of the optimization of the four elements of disease risk, intervention providers, intervention means, and intervention timing, respectively.

Chapter 2 is Surgical Risk Management: there are five sections. Section 1 reviews the brief history of surgical development and helps to recognize the surgical risks that have occurred in history, been solved, and have not been solved. Section 2 clarifies the theory of surgical risk control and details the composition and framework of surgical risk control system. From Section 3 to Section 5, according to the logical sequence of surgical risk pre-control system, the risk management is introduced in detail from three aspects: risk identification, risk evaluation, and risk intervention.

Chapter 3 is Decision-Making Process for Interveners: there are five sections. Section 1 details the classification, characteristics, and influencing factors of clinical decision-making. Section 2 focuses on the process from diagnostic decision-making to therapeutic decision-making, as well as the quality needed to cultivate clinical thinking. Section 3 introduces how to use evidence-based medicine in decision-making and its important impact on intervention provider decision-making. Section 4 introduces the MDT model into intervention provider decision-making, extends individual intervention provider decision-making to the level of multidisciplinary consultation, and demonstrates the importance of MDT through specific clinical cases.

Chapter 4 is Optimization of Interventions: a total of four sections. Section 1 details the characteristics, classification, and clinical significance of intervention optimization from the perspective of damage control with specific examples. Section 2 focuses on the driving effect of theoretical innovation on the optimization of intervention means. Section 3 introduces how to simplify and standardize the diagnosis and treatment process through the pathing, patterning, and modularization of intervention means, which is conducive to improving the overall level of intervention. Section 4 introduces in detail how to optimize the means of intervention and the effective allocation of medical resources from the perspective of cost-effectiveness optimization. Section 5 closely follows the pace of scientific and technological development, focuses on the development status of artificial intelligence in the medical field, and puts forward new requirements for how to promote the development of artificial intelligence in the medical field, which helps to better use artificial intelligence and other informatization technologies.

Chapter 5 is The choice of intervention timing: a total of three sections. This chapter focuses on the concept of intervention timing. From Section 1 to Section 3, we elaborate on how to grasp the optimal combination of disease risk, intervention providers, intervention means, and intervention timing to achieve the best intervention timing choice through six specific clinical examples from the perspective of disease risk, intervention providers, and intervention tools, respectively.

Chapter 6 is Strategies of clinical decision-making for improving prognosis: a total of four sections. This chapter applies the concept of prognosis control surgery to surgical practice and summarizes the four core strategies of bleeding control, approach, resection, and reconstruction, each of which is specifically explained by 1–2 clinical cases.

In order to adapt to the rapid development of medical science and technology, promote the timely update of the concept of surgical diagnosis and treatment, realize the whole process of optimal prognosis for patients, so that patients can obtain the best therapeutic effect, we propose the theory of prognosis control surgery and complete this monograph. This monograph can be used as a reference and study for clinicians and medical students in the field of surgery and will be beneficial in developing a holistic view of surgical diagnosis and treatment as well as improving the prognosis of patients.

Introduction of Editors

Chief Editor

Rong Liu

Deputy Editors

Qu Liu
Hongchen Ji
Ruiquan Zhou

Introduction

Current medical models include empirical medicine, which is dominated by the experience of the intervention provider, and evidence-based medicine, which relies on the choice of interventions. In the traditional empirical medicine model, doctors treat patients based on their own knowledge of diseases and clinical experience, and their medical quality relies on their experience and subjective decisions, which makes it difficult to grasp the scientificity and standardization of the treatment process and to control the results of treatment and patient prognosis. Evidence-based medicine emphasizes that medical decision-making must be based on the results of clinical studies with high evidence levels to reduce the impact of subjective factors of doctors on the diagnosis and treatment of diseases through objective evidence. However, evidence-based medicine attaches too much importance to the selection of intervention means and lacks the evaluation of the ability and experience of intervention providers, which is easy to cause the phenomenon that intervention providers cannot fully master a certain intervention means.

With the arrival of the Internet and big data era, informatization technology represented by artificial intelligence is more and more widely used in the medical field, and new disease diagnosis and treatment methods emerge in endlessly. These high-tech diagnosis and treatment methods bring not only simple advanced diagnosis and treatment methods to medicine but also challenges to the diagnosis and treatment concept. In order to comply with the developmental changes of the times and technology, we have proposed a new concept of prognosis control surgery, which emphasizes the optimal prognosis and the best outcome for patients, makes full use of information technology such as artificial intelligence to reduce the uncertainty in the treatment process and the unevenness of the treatment level, and selects the most appropriate intervention means and intervention timing through objective intervention provider evaluation to control the disease risk in advance to a minimum. We hope that surgical intervention providers can integrate the concept of prognosis control surgery into daily clinical practice, so that each patient can receive the most timely and effective treatment and obtain the best prognostic effect. At the same time, with the development of science and technology and the times, the concept of prognosis control is also continuously developing and improving. Readers are invited to criticize and correct it.

Faculty of Hepato-pancreato-biliary Surgery
Institute of Hepatobiliary Surgery of PLA
Chinese PLA General Hospital
Beijing, China
February 2019

Rong Liu

Contents

Introduction

1

Rong Liu and Qu Liu

Abstract

With the advent of network information technology and big data era and the continuous application of artificial intelligence and other information technologies in the medical field, the authors put forward the concept of prognosis control surgery according to the current situation of medical technology development and the direction of modern medical development and elaborated on four aspects of disease risk management, requirements of interveners, optimization of interventions, and selection of intervention timing, respectively.

1 Introduction to Clinical Decision-Making for Improving Prognosis

Traditional medical research is based on empirical medicine, and physicians diagnose and treat patients based on their own perception of the disease and non-experimental clinical experience. At this stage, the physician's competence and experience are considered to be the main factors influencing the patient's prognosis. The limitations of the era of empirical medicine are obvious, the quality of diagnosis and treatment depends too much on the experience accumulation of physicians and subjective real-time decision-making, the scientificity and standardization of the diagnosis and treatment process are difficult to grasp, and the results of treatment and patient prognosis are difficult to control.

With the reflection on empirical medicine and the deepening of clinical research guided by statistics, some scholars put forward the concept of evidence-based medicine in the middle and late twentieth century and made evidence-based medicine

R. Liu (✉) · Q. Liu
Faculty of Hepato-pancreato-biliary Surgery, Chinese PLA General Hospital, Beijing, China

R. Liu (ed.), *Clinical Decision Making for Improving Prognosis*,
https://doi.org/10.1007/978-981-19-2952-6_1

assume the task of guiding medical decision-making. In practice, evidence-based medicine emphasizes that medical decisions must be based on the results of clinical studies with high levels of evidence, while considering the subjective needs of patients, the purpose of which is to reduce the impact of subjective factors of physicians on the diagnosis and treatment of diseases through objective evidence. In the concept of evidence-based medicine, diagnosis and treatment decisions and interventions replace intervention providers and become the main factors to control disease risk and affect prognosis. The emergence of evidence-based medicine has promoted the progress of medical research and the overall improvement of medical level to a certain extent, but it attaches too much importance to the selection of intervention means while ignoring the evaluation of the ability and experience of intervention providers.

With the arrival of the era of Internet and big data, with the application of artificial intelligence and other information technologies in the medical field, advanced disease diagnosis and treatment methods emerge in endlessly, and traditional medical treatment dominated by the experience of intervention providers and evidence-based medicine relying excessively on intervention means have been newly impacted and challenged.

1.1 Concept and Characteristics of Prognosis Control Surgery

According to the current development situation of medical science and technology and the development direction of modern medicine, we put forward the concept of prognosis control surgery: using artificial intelligence and other information technology, predicting the risk of surgical diseases, formulating reasonable intervention objectives, selecting the best intervention provider, intervention means, intervention timing and their best combination, and controlling, realizing the whole process of optimal prognosis, so that patients can get the best outcome, referred to as prognosis control surgery. Prognosis control surgery emphasizes the combination of artificial intelligence technology on the basis of traditional medical diagnosis and treatment methods to control the risk of surgical diseases by exploring the optimal combination of intervention providers, intervention means, and intervention timing and finally realize the optimal prognosis of patients. The theory of prognosis control surgery provides a key idea for the development of new disease diagnosis and treatment strategies and patient prognosis model analysis, constituting the basic framework of disease risk control theory. Prognosis control surgery is the product of combining the latest medical development technology and concept with the existing medical system, reflecting the clinical need to continuously improve the diagnosis and treatment effect and maximize the benefits of patients. Intervention providers can only achieve the most efficient risk management of disease and optimal patient prognosis by integrating the concept of prognosis control surgery into all aspects of clinical care.

We refer here to the concept of intervention providers, and what is an intervention provider? The implementation process of medical treatment is not only the diagnosis and treatment process of attending physicians, but also includes the medical related personnel including anesthesiologists, nurses, technicians, and even accompanying personnel. In the clinical process, the role of physicians cannot be only emphasized. All the personnel related to this medical treatment are intervention providers. The behavior, operation, and decision of these intervention providers may have an impact on the rehabilitation and health of patients. For example, even if the surgeon is highly qualified and skilled, the surgery cannot be carried out without the cooperation of a good anesthesiologist. Without the cooperation and support of a good nursing team, it is difficult for the patient to recover smoothly after a difficult operation. We often encounter the situation that young physicians consult experienced nurses and even attendants in clinical practice. The clinical knowledge and experience are sometimes unable to go to school in books and require the accumulation of touching and rolling in practice for a long time.

The integration of prognosis control surgery into clinical diagnosis and treatment requires grasping three key characteristics: (1) the ultimate goal of prognosis control surgery is to achieve the best prognosis of patients, and the prognosis of patients is not only the primary goal of medical intervention, but also the only evaluation criteria; (2) the realization process of prognosis control surgery is actually the risk management process of the disease, that is, the process of identifying risks, assessing risks, and controlling risks; (3) the optimization and combination of intervention providers, intervention means, and intervention timing are the means of realization, and the optimal control of risks and the best prognosis of patients are achieved through the continuous optimization and configuration of the three factors of intervention (Fig. 1.1).

1.2 Prognosis of Patient Is the Ultimate Goal

The progress of science and technology is a strong impetus to promote the continuous progress and development of medicine. With the continuous upgrading of technology and equipment, continuous update of diagnosis and treatment methods and continuous improvement of medical concepts, intervention providers will be able to realize more reasonable clinical decisions and better benefit patients. However, at present, the research on medicine seems to be excessively focused on the technology and equipment itself, and even sometimes for the application of new technologies and new businesses, ignoring what benefits such doing can bring to patients, the situation of treatment for treatment and surgery for surgery, ignoring the fundamental purpose of the development of medical science and technology is to improve the quality of disease treatment and improve the prognosis of patients.

Patient prognosis is the most important criterion to judge the quality of medical intervention, and optimal patient prognosis is a goal that should always be adhered to in the treatment of diseases. With the more and more detailed division of medical subspecialties as well as more and more diverse selection of treatment means, the treatment means specialized by different physicians are becoming more and more alienated. Although the choice of the treatment that is good at itself can improve the

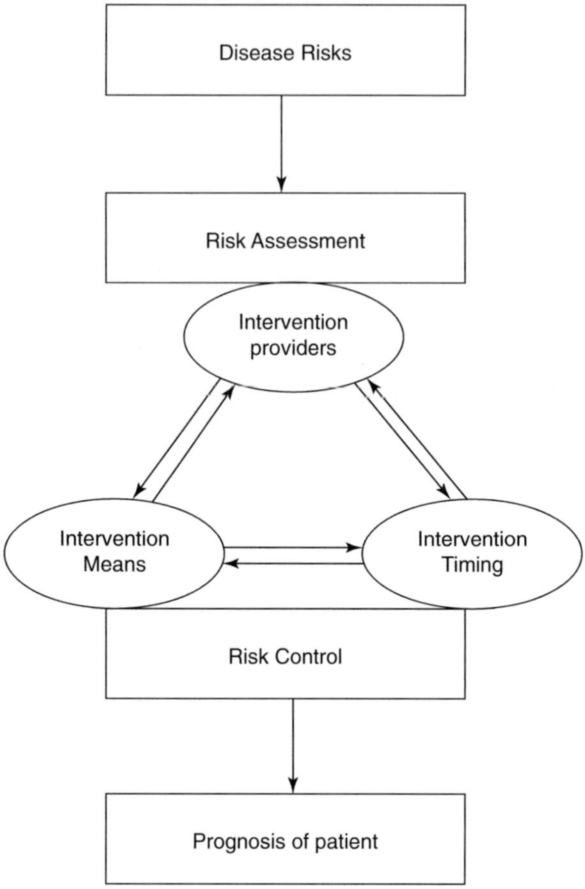

Fig. 1.1 Flowchart of prognosis control surgery

quality of treatment to a certain extent, the nature of the treatment itself determines the margin and upper limit of its efficacy, and in the face of different patients, the factors of its own ability become the shackle of the choice of treatment. It is an essential quality for excellent physicians to take the patient's prognosis as the fundamental orientation and select the appropriate specialty, physician, and treatment.

1.3 The Management of Disease Risks Is the Realization Process

Disease risk refers to the combination of the possibility of an adverse event caused by a disease and its consequences. There are three characteristics of disease risk: (1) multiple risks of a single disease may not be independent of each other. (2) There can be a dynamic transformation between the different risks of a single disease. (3) There is a dynamic correlation between disease risk and interventions. Judging from the theory of prognosis control surgery, the prognosis of patients is the ultimate goal pursued by medical behavior, and the process of medical behavior should be the process of seeking disease risk minimization, that is, the intervention provider exchanges the minimum intervention risk for the maximum disease risk optimization. We refer to the optimization of disease risk during intervention as risk management in the theory of prognostic surgery, and the process of implementing prognosis control surgery is the risk management process of diseases.

The risk management process is divided into two parts: risk assessment and risk control. The scope of risk assessment shall be comprehensive and specific, including the possible risks caused by disease factors, intervention providers, means, and intervention timing. In the process of risk assessment, it shall be noted that disease risk, intervention provider risk, risk of intervention means, and risk of intervention timing do not exist independently, but are interconnected, interact with each other, and even transform each other. For example, incorrect diagnosis and treatment decisions and irrational use of intervention means by intervention providers for diseases may increase the risk of intervention, and inappropriate intervention timing may also bring additional risk of intervention. And excellent intervention providers are able to reduce the risk of intervention means and intervention timing within their own ability, thereby maximizing the control of disease risk.

The process of risk control is the core operation process of prognosis control surgery, which is the process for the intervention provider to select the appropriate intervention timing to implement the optimization and combination of intervention means. In order to realize the optimal risk control, it is necessary not only to comprehensively master the traditional medical methods, but also to closely follow the frontiers of discipline development and apply the informatization method represented by advanced artificial intelligence into the diagnosis and treatment process, so as to improve the intelligence, standardization, and automation degree of surgical practice, change the diagnosis and treatment mode of surgical diseases, and change the thinking mode of surgeons. The main purpose of risk control is to realize the balance between disease risk, intervention risk, and patient benefit, carry out repeated risk evaluation under the principle of ensuring the maximum benefit of patients, and try to realize the optimal prognosis of patients through the continuous optimization and configuration combination of intervention providers, intervention means, and intervention timing.

1.4 The Optimal Combination of the Three Factors of Intervention Is a Means of Realization

Intervention providers, intervention means, and intervention timing cover all aspects of disease risk management and are also the three most important factors affecting the prognosis of patient. These three factors interact and influence each other. In the prognosis control surgery, it is necessary to consider the three factors together, so as to realize the optimization and reasonable combination of intervention provider, intervention means, and intervention timing, so as to realize the maximum benefit for patients.

Intervention providers are the main body of the diagnosis and treatment process, and the experience and ability of intervention providers determine the formulation of clinical decisions, determine the choice of intervention timing, and also determine the quality of the implementation of intervention means. As the leader and executor of prognosis control surgery, intervention providers need to have the scientific and rigorous spirit of medical practitioners and also need to keep pace with the times and continuously innovate in the development of medical science and technology and intelligent medicine. In addition to improving the ability of clinical thinking and judgment from a large number of clinical practices, intervention providers should also be good at using evidence-based medicine, multidisciplinary collaboration, big data and artificial intelligence and other intervention means to improve the accuracy of clinical decision-making, improve the effectiveness of surgical intervention, and improve the timeliness of intervention timing. Since the object of medical work is people rather than only abstract diseases, intervention providers also need to relate the patient's emotions, improve the patient's treatment experience and psychological needs through adequate humanistic care, and improve the therapeutic effect of diseases.

Intervention is a direct tool to complete disease intervention, and reasonable selection and appropriate use of intervention is a key factor to achieve a good prognosis for patients. The current development of medical science and technology is mainly reflected in the enrichment and progress of intervention means, which not only realizes the upgrading of existing diagnosis and treatment methods, but also brings more innovative diagnosis and treatment means and concepts. However, the update of equipment, technology, and method is only the surface phenomenon of scientific and technological development. Whether science and technology can be better used and whether it can be better combined with the diagnosis and treatment of diseases requires the innovation of intervention concept to realize the minimization of intervention risks, damage control, simplification of complex surgery and minimally invasive surgery and realize the optimization of cost-effectiveness.

The intervention timing is a time node for the intervention provider to apply the intervention to control and intervene in disease risk. The intervention timing is a subjective factor of "invisible and untouchable" in the medical process, and there is a close internal link between it and other elements. The choice of intervention timing is not only affected by disease risk, intervention provider, and intervention means, but also can act backwards on disease risk and affect the effect of intervention and the prognosis of patients. Appropriate intervention timing contributes to the achievement of intervention goals, while at the wrong intervention timing, even the optimal combination of intervention providers and interventions often fails to achieve a good prognosis. In clinical work, the intervention providers need to judge the relationship between intervention risks and intervention benefits in real time. If the intervention risks are higher than the intervention benefits, the intervention cannot be implemented. The intervention timing is not static. When the risk of disease and the corresponding intervention providers and intervention means change, the selection of intervention timing should also be adjusted accordingly, that is, the dynamic optimization of intervention timing. Dynamic optimization of intervention timing requires intervention providers to be able to flexibly grasp the intervention timing and be co-ordinators of clinical intervention, rather than mechanical executors, and intervention providers are good at thinking, comprehensively grasp various elements of prognosis control medicine, and carry out reasonable allocation and optimization combination.

Due to the different medical education background and work platform, there are great differences between the abilities and experiences of intervention providers, and the mastery of intervention means and the grasp of intervention timing vary. The existing medical model overemphasizes the selection of intervention means with high evidence level, ignores whether the intervention provider can master this technology and method, lacks the assessment of the intervention provider's own experience and professional ability, and easily enters the misunderstanding that the intervention provider and intervention means cannot match. For the first time, the ability and state of the intervention provider are included in the evaluation system in the prognosis control surgery. Through the third-party perspective, based on the intervention provider's mastery of different intervention means and emotional state, the intervention means and intervention timing are more objectively and effectively selected. In addition, the rapid development of informatization technologies such as machine learning, image recognition, and artificial intelligence represented by intraoperative navigation not only promotes the continuous optimization of intervention means, but also puts forward higher requirements for intervention providers. Intervention providers need to keep pace with the times, adjust the diagnosis and treatment concept, apply new intervention means to the intervention process, and develop the corresponding intervention timing in order to achieve the optimal combination of the three factors of intervention. Moreover, with the further development of artificial intelligence, with the closer and closer human–computer interaction, the machine will continuously realize the expert empowerment, gradually change from the intervention means to the intervention provider with judgment and operation ability, while the human originally as the intervention provider will become the supervisor of the intervention process.

Prognosis control surgery is an innovative medical concept based on the great progress of basic science and medical technology. Its purpose is to make medical intervention adapt to the new technical environment, exert the maximum efficiency of new technologies and methods, and obtain the maximum benefit for patients. Prognosis control surgery can guide the formulation and implementation of clinical decisions in a complex diagnosis and treatment process. Through a complete set of perfect theoretical system and implementation methods, prognosis control surgery can maximize the benefits of patients from all stages of the disease and from all aspects of disease intervention. Prognosis control surgery also needs to be continuously developed and improved, keep pace with the times, adapt to the rapid development of medical science and technology, meet the growing treatment needs of patients, and better use the achievements of scientific and technological development to serve patients.

2 Disease Risk Management

The core of prognosis control surgery is to measure the impact of the interaction between the intervention provider, the intervention means, and the intervention timing on the risk of disease with the goal of optimal patient prognosis. The process is also the process of balancing the risk of disease with the risk of intervention and the benefit of intervention and can be called the risk management process. In simple terms, risk management includes risk assessment and risk intervention. Risk assessment is implemented before intervention, with the purpose of selecting the best intervention provider and intervention means through the identification and evaluation of disease risks, while risk intervention is implemented during intervention, with the purpose of avoiding or limiting the risks during intervention through the advance control of disease risks. Effective risk management helps to control disease risk, optimize the intervention process, and reduce damage to patients.

2.1 The Concept of Disease Risk Management

Patient prognosis is the ultimate aim pursued by medical behavior and the only criterion to evaluate the quality of medical interventions. The process of medical behavior should be one that seeks to minimize the risk of disease, in which the intervention providers play a leading role. Evidence-based medicine is a major advance in the medical research concept, but limited by technical conditions and research methods, evidence-based medicine does not have the conditions to consider intervention providers. The development and progress of artificial intelligence, big data, Internet, and other technologies make it possible to consider the interaction between intervention providers and disease risk, intervention means, and intervention timing in current medical behaviors. In the process of disease intervention (treatment), the intervention providers reduce the risk of disease through the intervention means, but the means of implementing the intervention similarly bring new intervention risks. The patient benefit in the medical process is expressed in Fig. 1.2.

The goal of medical care should be to maximize patient benefit by exchanging the minimum risk of intervention for the maximum risk reduction of disease. When the risks of the intervention outweigh the benefits of the intervention, it is a gain or loss for the patient. For example, in the treatment of hepatic hemangiomas >5 cm, many doctors prefer surgical resection, while patients and their families are often willing to choose surgical resection even if there are no symptoms due to fear of

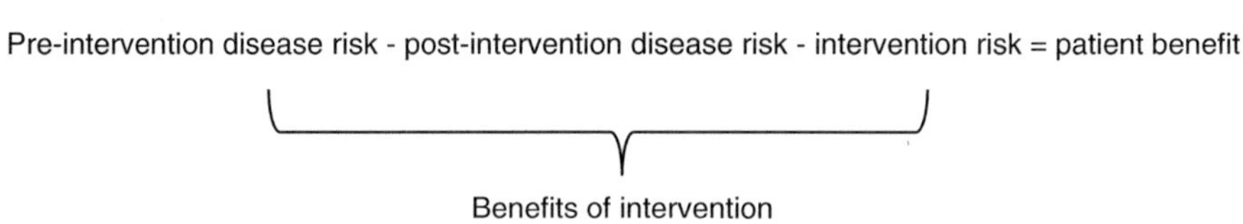

Fig. 1.2 The patient benefit in the medical process

"tumors." However, in the follow-up of 63.2 months by Giuliante et al., less than 20% (14 cases) of 74 patients with hepatic hemangioma had increased tumor size, while spontaneous hemorrhage of hepatic hemangioma accounted for no more than 1%. In this case, the risk of hepatic resection has exceeded the disease risk of hepatic hemangioma itself, the benefit of intervention will not outweigh the risk of intervention, and the patient benefit is calculated to be negative. Therefore, for asymptomatic or mildly symptomatic hepatic hemangioma with tumor diameter >5 cm, follow-up observation can be recommended, or hepatic artery embolization therapy, radiofrequency ablation, and other means with less risk of intervention can be selected to improve the benefits of patients and avoid the overpayment of intervention.

The core idea of the above decision-making process is to balance the relationship between the benefits of the intervention and the risks of the intervention, and the patient is considered to have the greatest benefit when the difference between the two is the largest. Under the premise that the disease risk before intervention is difficult to control, it can be considered that the smaller the intervention risk, the smaller the disease risk after intervention, and the more beneficial the patient. We refer to the optimization of disease risk in the process of surgical diagnosis and treatment as the risk management in the prognosis control surgical theory, the ultimate purpose of which is to maximize the benefits of patients and improve the prognosis of patients. The core idea is to balance the relationship between the risks of intervention and the benefits of intervention, in an attempt to exchange the minimum risk of intervention for the maximum benefits of patients. The specific implementation process can be divided into two parts: risk assessment and risk intervention.

2.2 Basic Ideas and Processes for Risk Assessment

In the risk assessment process, risk identification shall be performed first. The contents of risk identification include disease risks, intervention providers, and possible risks brought by intervention means. The identification range shall be comprehensive and specific. The risk of a disease includes the symptoms, signs, functional decompensation, organ failure, and even death that the disease may bring to the patients. The risk of an intervention provider includes the risks that may be caused by the techniques, experience, emotion, control ability of the intervention means, and other factors. The risk of an intervention means includes the risks that may be caused by different treatment methods, means, and techniques. The risk of an intervention timing includes the direction that may be caused by different intervention timing.

After comprehensive risk identification, the identified risks need to be evaluated In the process of risk evaluation, it shall be noted that the risks in the above four aspects are not independent, but interrelated, mutual influence and interaction, and the change in the risk in a certain aspect may lead to the change in the risks in the other two aspects or even the whole process of diagnosis and treatment. For surgical treatment of pancreatic cancer, the interaction between the intervention (surgery) and disease risk (pancreatic cancer) may lead to increased risk of diseases after intervention, such as incision infection, pancreatic fistula, abdominal bleeding, bile leakage, gastrointestinal dysfunction, etc. The interaction between the intervention provider, the intervention means, and the disease risk is generally reflected in the different control abilities of the intervention provider for the disease intervention experience and the intervention means. For example, if an intervention provider is more familiar with and experienced in the treatment of gastrointestinal diseases, but lacks the treatment experience for liver diseases, it can be considered that the intervention risk of the interaction between the intervention provider and gastrointestinal diseases is greater than that of the interaction with liver diseases. Studying the interaction between intervention providers and disease risk is particularly important in the context of the increasingly refined division of medical subspecialties. For example, general surgery is initially a specialty, and with the further deepening of the understanding of disease risk, it has differentiated into multiple subspecialties such as hepatobiliary and pancreatic, gastrointestinal, thyromammary, and vascular, and even subspecialties of liver surgery and pancreatic surgery. At this point, a surgeon has been unable to be proficient in all diseases within the general surgery specialty and may only make a difference in one direction. There are very few "perfect intervention providers" who are significantly proficient in these multiple subdivisions at the same time, and more intervention providers will choose a certain branch and a specific disease as the main research direction, which is an inevitable trend of increasing understanding of the disease.

The relationship between intervention providers and intervention means is the same. In the form of continuous progress and diversification of intervention means, fewer and fewer intervention providers will be proficient in all intervention means of a subspecialty, and more and more intervention providers will be more and more proficient in a certain intervention means instead. For example, the earliest hepatobiliary surgery was completed by laparotomy. By the 1990s, with the rapid development of laparoscopic techniques, laparoscopic techniques were gradually carried out in cholecystectomy, hepatectomy, and pancreatectomy, resulting in surgeons specializing in laparoscopic surgery. In the past decade, with the comprehensive optimization of laparoscopic surgery by robotic surgical systems in terms of three-dimensional imaging and fine operation, the scope of application of robotic surgery has become more and more extensive, so the corresponding robotic surgeons have emerged. Therefore, in the process of risk evaluation, the disease risk, intervention provider, intervention means and their interaction should be considered and carefully evaluated.

Risk evaluation is the core process of risk assessment, and its process shall be repeatedly evaluated in accordance with the principle of maximizing the benefits of patients, that is, to select the intervention means with the greatest difference between the benefits of intervention and the risks of intervention within the optional range of patients. It should be noted that if the benefits of the intervention from all intervention providers/intervention combinations cannot outweigh the risks of the intervention, termination of the intervention should be chosen. The process of typical risk assessment can be simplified as shown in Fig. 1.3.

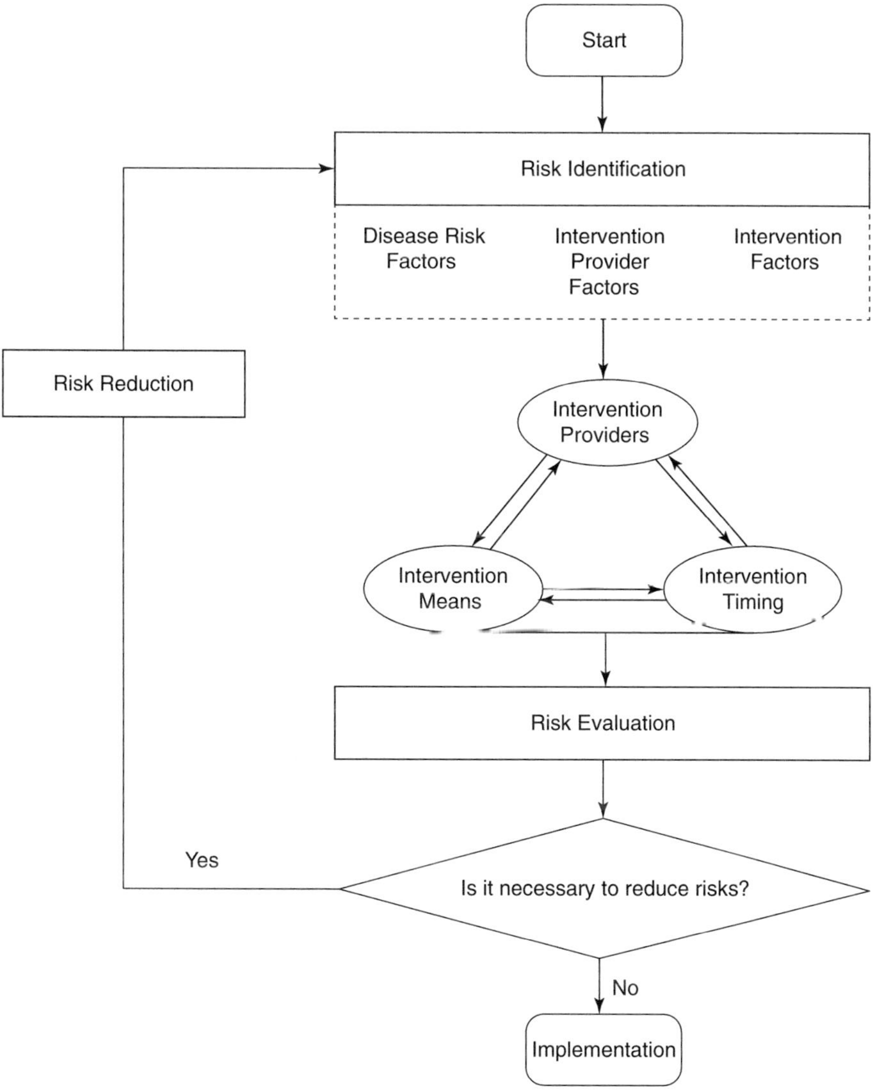

Fig. 1.3 Typical Risk Assessment Process

2.3 Basic Ideas and Processes of Risk Intervention

Risk prevention is the preventive measures taken before a risk occurs, and its goal is to reduce the incidence of surgical risks or the degree of injury of adverse consequences. Risk prevention is based on risk identification, risk evaluation, and other early risk pre-control measures to effectively prevent the evaluated, possible disease risks and intervention risks. Risk prevention is mainly implemented before the occurrence of risk, that is, "prior" measures, which are intended to reduce the incidence or degree of risk by changing the main factors leading to risk, changing the risk environment, and interrupting the downstream chain of risk factors.

Risk control refers to the degree that clinical intervention providers actively and consciously take intervention means to control risk events and reduce the adverse consequences during the intervention. When risk control is taken, the risk has not occurred, and its fundamental purpose is to reach the expectation of risk assessment, reduce the degree of injury and prevent the further development of risk. Risk control can effectively control the degree of damage caused by risks from the sources causing risks and prevent the subsequent risk cascade.

In fact, risk control is a kind of countermeasures in advance, aiming at risk accidents, adverse consequences, and various losses, quickly formulate countermeasures and implement actions, so as to reduce the severity of adverse consequences caused by risks and maximize the protection of patients' interests. Risk control refers to pre-response, rather than post-remedial measures, which have been taken in advance, but can only play a role in the intervention process. Risk control is a sequential and unified "active attack" process that aims to reduce the consequences caused by risks. For example, when removing a tumor invading the vein, we usually free the distal and proximal veins and preset the blocking band, which aims to quickly and effectively control bleeding once the vein is injured during surgery causing massive hemorrhage. For another example, in order to effectively control bleeding during hepatectomy, if the main blood supply vessels and communicating branch vessels in the precut area can be controlled in advance, the risk of bleeding can be actively grasped during surgery to make it easy.

It is divided into three levels according to the severity and controllability of the consequences caused by the risk (Fig. 1.4).

The first level is mandatory risk control. The risk at this level has the most serious consequences and can be controlled by the intervention provider following procedures. For example, during surgery, severe bleeding and heart failure can directly lead to patient death, so preoperative blood preparation and cardiopulmonary function evaluation are required to avoid them; for another example, the counting and verification of drugs and devices in medical behaviors also belong to the category of mandatory risk control. These avoidance processes are less difficult and are usually supervised by regulations or industry practices, which are the most basic requirements for risk control.

The second level is technical risk control. Risk consequences at this level are severe and can be controlled by professional training for most intervention providers. For example, the surgeon and assistant should be familiar with the surgical procedure and the basic operation required according to their respective responsibilities to avoid the increased risk of intervention caused by unskilled or irregular operation. Technical risk control is usually implemented without mandatory standard supervision, but it is generally considered to be a technical content that must be mastered by specialists after training.

The third level is empirical risk control. Risk at this level has predictable consequences and needs to be controlled by experienced intervention providers. For

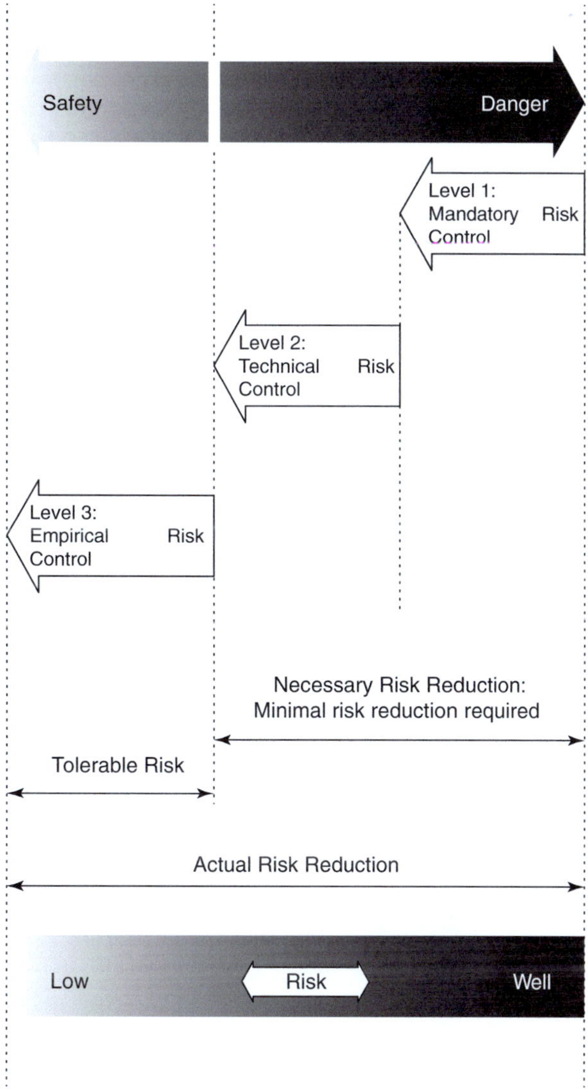

Fig. 1.4 Level of Risk Control

example, the quality of pancreaticojejunostomy is a key factor in determining whether pancreatic fistula bleeding occurs after pancreaticoduodenectomy. Pancreatic fistula bleeding rates reported by pancreatic surgery centers vary widely, which is directly related to the experience of intervention providers in the management of pancreaticojejunostomy. Some scholars believe that pancreatic surgery centers with less than 20 cases of pancreaticoduodenectomy performed annually are not suitable for such surgery. Thus, empirical risk control is more common in difficult intervention processes, while there are often controversies in implementation methods.

Generally, technical risk control is the minimum standard required for the intervention process. Risk reduction by mandatory and technical risk control is called risk reduction necessary and is a general requirement in medical behavior. Therefore, in the process of risk management, it is necessary to ensure that the combination of intervention provider and intervention means can realize the requirements for technical risk control at least. The third level of risk control is difficult to make clear requirements because the scope of implementation is limited to experienced intervention providers. The characteristics determine that it has the largest optimizable space, is an important component of risk management, and is closely related to patient prognosis. The risk reduction achieved by the three levels together is the actual risk reduction during the intervention.

3 Knowledge and Experience of Interveners

In the process of intervention, human is the core factor, making decisions depends on human, grasping the timing depends on human, implementing intervention also depends on human, human knowledge, technology, thought, morality, and style of work play a very important role in the process of intervention. Patients depend on each other for life, and this trust is both stress and impetus for intervention providers. However, due to the differences in their upbringing and opportunities, the technical ability and experience of intervention providers also vary greatly. To become an excellent intervention provider, in addition to the pursuit of excellent technology, it is necessary to fully improve self-cultivation, to achieve both virtue and talent, and to unite knowledge and practice in order to be comfortable and calm in the clinical treatment process.

3.1 Humanistic Care

Humanistic care is the embodiment of the core spirit and value orientation of medicine. The object of medical work is human rather than abstract diseases. In addition to biological diseases, patients will also have many disorders in psychology and sociology. The purpose of medicine is therefore not only the treatment of disease, but also the care and attention of the patients. This requires clinicians to pay attention to the change of bio-psycho-social medical model, not only to the disease itself, but also to patients and to the psychological and humanistic needs of patients. Excellent intervention providers must treat diseases and relieve symptoms at the same time, more through empathy and comfort of patients' emotional behavior, to help patients relieve, release, and enlighten the psychological problems such as restlessness and anxiety in the heart, in order to obtain good clinical results. If the intervention provider only considers the pure biological needs of diagnosing and treating the disease, does not consider the psychological status and social environment of the patient, and cannot listen to the psychological and sociological needs of the patient, then medical work is often difficult to achieve because it is not cooperated by the patient.

"To cure sometime, to relieve often, to comfort always," Dr. Trudeau's epitaph not only reflects the limitations of medicine, but also shows the universality and importance of humanistic care and psychological counseling in medical treatment. However, due to the limitations of medical development, the field of medical technology is limited, and there is always a place beyond the reach of medicine, such as hepatitis B, an infectious chronic disease, which has a long course of disease, is easy to relapse and is infectious, and patients often experience different degrees of tension and restlessness and even lead to the aggravation of the disease. Patients with advanced cancer have more psychological anxiety and fear in addition to physical pain, and this mental affliction is even greater than physical pain. In this case, the intervention providers need to strengthen the attention to humanistic care, emphasize that medical treatment is patient-centered rather than disease-centered, multi-empathy, improve the doctor–patient communication and psychological counseling to the medical level, and run through and integrate the idea of humanistic care into the drip of clinical work in the diagnosis and treatment process.

The father of medicine, Hippocrates, once said that "doctors have three magic weapons, the first is language, the second is drugs, and the third is scalpels." Qiu Fazu, the father of surgery in China, always warmed up the stethoscope before using it, always waited in the consultation room in advance for each outpatient visit, and personally replied to every letter from patients. He demonstrates humanistic care in every clinical detail. In the medical process, active humanistic care can mobilize the positive factors of patients, relieve psychological hidden dangers, enhance the confidence to overcome the disease, so that they actively cooperate with the treatment and better promote the rehabilitation of the disease. If the humanistic characteristics of medicine are removed, it is to abandon the essential attributes of medicine, and it is difficult to heal the psychological trauma of patients even if the disease is cured.

A survey has shown that nearly half of medical disputes are caused by lack of communication between medical staff and patients, rather than problems in medical level. During the intervention, the intervention provider needs to perceive the patient's emotions and pressures, explain the possible causes and the next examination and treatment plan as far as possible, understand and respect the wishes and choices of the patient and his family through full communication with the patient and his family, use his professional knowledge to guide and obtain the trust of the patient, construct a relatively easy medical environment and atmosphere, and lay the foundation for further treatment.

3.2 Putting Virtue First

Qiu Fazu, the father of surgery in China, said, "Those whose virtue is not close to Buddha cannot be doctors," which requires doctors to be both virtuous and talented, with virtue as the first priority. When confronted with a difficult and complex case, it is a test of an intervention provider's "virtue" whether he or she thinks first of benefiting the patient or first of protecting himself or herself. The risk of treatment is greater, the greater the risk the intervention provider takes. For the same patient at the same risk, why some doctors dare to do the surgery, while others are afraid to do it? This is not only related to the ability and knowledge of doctors, but also closely related to the "morality" of doctors. Only with great determination there can be more methods, and the starting and ending points of the intervention providers are different, so the thinking process and the results of implementation are naturally different.

Of course this is not to encourage intervention providers to treat for treatment and operate for surgery. There are indeed such doctors in clinical practice, in order to complete difficult surgery or implement new technologies and new businesses, knowing that they may be invasive to patients, they should also complete the treatment beyond the indications, which is even more contrary to the principle of medical treatment and violates the moral original intention of healers. Our surgeons cannot take the completion of a difficult major surgery as the standard of treatment, cannot blindly pursue the time and number of surgery, but should take the control of injury, protection of function, saving lives as the primary task of treatment, reduce the invasiveness of surgery, avoid ineffective surgery in line with the requirements of the healer's benevolence. For example, how to grasp the conversion to laparotomy in the field of minimally invasive surgery? Sometimes doctors continue to complete the operation in order to avoid conversion to laparotomy, even if the intraoperative blood loss and organ injury have reached the level of conversion to laparotomy. They do not know that conversion to laparotomy in order to reduce the patient's trauma is a mature embodiment of surgeons and an embodiment of medical ethics. Therefore, whether the intervention provider enters or retreats under certain conditions? We must weigh the pros and cons and make rational clinical decisions centered on the patient's interests.

3.3 Be Diligent

In today's era of rapid development of science and technology, there has been a trend of more and more specialized and refined knowledge division, which will be conducive to the progress and development of various disciplines. However, the research object of medicine is the overall living people, rather than a mechanical part, and must not be diagnosed and treated with the idea of separation. High-level clinical intervention requires our clinical intervention providers to have a highly comprehensive idea, overcome the tubular thinking defects caused by too thin division through comprehensive knowledge accumulation and reserve, transform knowledge into clinical skills, and better serve the clinical practice. As the saying goes "A doctor should have celestial being's talent," only by diligently studying and learning multidisciplinary knowledge they can be well-rounded talents, and only by comprehensively improving their professional knowledge and business level they can make the right clinical decisions calmly in the face of emergency and critical situations.

Medicine is a specialty combining theory and practice. The medical theory separated from practice is only an empty talk and cannot treat patients. In addition to mastering basic clinical skills, intervention providers also need to achieve technical specialization, maintain the refinement and refining of skills in diligent study and hard practice, complete the update and reserve of professional technology in continuous practice, and gradually achieve versatility. The older generation of medical scientists often teaches us to be a "clinician" and not an "out of bed doctor." That is to say, only by going deep into the patient we can empathize with the patient's symptoms, notice subtle changes in signs, and improve intervention ability through the accumulation of experience.

To do a good job in clinical decision-making, it is also necessary to take the initiative to learn, keep pace with the times, and maintain the spirit of innovation at all times. Nowadays, we are in the era of "Internet +," "big data," and "artificial intelligence." With the massive application of digital com006Dunication, image transmission, and Internet technology in medicine, the academic exchange between regions and internationally is increasing, and the information content of medical development is increasing dramatically in the order of magnitude. The market inquiry of various new drugs and new therapies and the upgrading of high-tech medical devices have strongly promoted the progress of clinical diagnosis and treatment. All of these not only promote the development of medicine, but also force clinicians to learn diligently and consciously, widely involve in the knowledge of multiple subject frontiers, and actively strive for excellent therapeutic effects, so as to grow into a clinical intervention provider with both moral and talent. For example, in the past, only palliative treatment with chemotherapy or symptomatic treatment was available for unresectable locally advanced pancreatic cancer, but the latest LAPACT study showed that induction chemotherapy had a better disease control rate and surgical conversion rate for tumors. On the basis of fully grasping the latest progress in the subject field, the author's team selected the chemotherapy induction regimen through communication with the patients and their families so that a patient with locally advanced pancreatic cancer had the chance of surgery, and the patient had radical resection by pancreaticoduodenectomy combined with portal vein repair during surgery. It is well-known that pancreaticoduodenectomy is the most complex and difficult operation in abdominal surgery. The surgical process and postoperative management are full of unpredictable risks. Intraoperative combined portal vein wall repair is a great test for the professional technology and psychological quality of surgeons, and these require usually long-term hard training and experience accumulation. The success of this operation is no accident, fully reflecting the comprehensive professional knowledge of the intervention providers, the wide field of vision closely following the academic frontiers and the superb and superb surgical skills.

3.4 Good at Thinking

"Success depends on forethought." To make a reasonable and accurate intervention, we must learn to think and be good at thinking, be able to find out the logic of diagnosis from the complex clinical data and examination report, and be able to weigh the advantages and disadvantages from a variety of treatment options to select the best treatment. This is why it is said that there is no intervention without thinking, and that prognosis control surgery requires the intervention provider to have a rational way of thinking and a logical mode of thinking. Medicine is a subject fraught with risks, and any clinical intervention has relative risks. Intervention providers need to have a clear understanding and judgment of possible risks and how to avoid them before implementing the intervention. In the process of intervention, only by mastering the mechanism, principle, and influencing factors of risks and doing a good job in the assessment and control of risks, risks can be effectively avoided and the initiative of intervention be grasped. What kind of risks do intervention providers need to think about when implementing an intervention? How likely is the risk to occur? How severe is the result of this risk? What is the effective way to respond? How well can the intervention provider and the patient withstand the risks? Only with prediction, plan, and prognosis control the smooth implementation and completion of diagnosis and treatment can be ensured.

In clinic, it is often encountered that the results of various examinations vary greatly from one another or even contradict each other. How to screen and integrate these intricate data is not only a professional problem, but also a problem of thinking methods. Clinicians should apply their professional knowledge combined with scientific thinking methods to analyze the examination data comprehensively, remove the falsehoods, and remove the essence, in order to achieve the purpose of clarifying the cause and effect, distinguishing the main and secondary, and removing the falsehoods and keeping the truth. For example, in the diagnosis of pancreatic tumors, the specificity and sensitivity of the examination method should be analyzed first, and the examination method with high specificity and sensitivity should be selected as far as possible. Contrast-enhanced MRI is certainly superior to MRI in the diagnosis of pancreatic tumors. Second, to analyze the limitations of the examination method itself, for example, the diagnosis of pancreatic tumors by B ultrasound may be interfered by flatulence. Finally, we should also be good at analyzing and comparing the similarities and differences of several imaging examination results and confirm each other with clinical symptoms. For example, in the diagnosis of pancreatic islet cell tumor, it is often encountered that MRI and CT cannot confirm the diagnosis or even find the tumor. Combined with the special clinical symptoms of hypoglycemia and the application of ultrasound, it may point out the direction for the diagnosis and treatment of tumors.

The accuracy of the choice of intervention means is directly related to the improvement of disease treatment and medical quality and to the rehabilitation and safety of patients. In the face of intricate and ever-changing diseases, how to make rapid and reasonable decisions from various alternative treatment options is an important indicator to measure the clinical workability of doctors. First of all, it is necessary to make overall plans and give consideration to it, focus on it, find the key links of the disease, grasp the main contradictions affecting the rehabilitation of patients at present, and formulate targeted treatment decisions. In the implementation process, it is necessary to pay attention to the main contradiction in the process of continuous transformation and timely adjust the plan to grasp the new main contradiction. Therefore, in the process of clinical diagnosis and treatment, we should be diligent in thinking, grasp the characteristics and development trend of the disease, review the situation, continuously adjust the diagnosis and treatment plan according to the development and change of the disease, and select the optimal and most feasible clinical decision from the interests of patients.

3.5 Emotional Control

The so-called emotional control is that the intervention provider can control his/her mood and cannot be interfered by environmental and human factors. The object of intervention is people, and the implementer of intervention is also people, so surgical intervention is not only a rational and calm thinking and analysis process, but usually emotional factors play a role in it and will be affected by social, cultural, and psychological factors to varying degrees. In sudden medical emergencies, the intervention provider is required to make a decisive scientific judgment of the clinical phenomenon, which often includes a variety of interfering factors in this situation, such as noisy environment, changes in the emotions of the physicians involved, patients and families, and various references from superior and subordinate physicians, making the sudden medical event more difficult to judge and handle. In addition to the accumulation of usual knowledge and clinical thinking training, the emotional control of doctors plays a key role in clinical decision-making. For example, postoperative abdominal bleeding is often sudden and rapid, and patients and their families will experience tension or even accompanying impatience and panic due to this sudden bleeding, which will adversely affect the doctor's clinical judgment and treatment decisions. At this time, it is necessary for clinical intervention providers to control their own emotions, eliminate the interference from themselves and external factors, and quickly judge whether the bleeding comes from the vascular stump or anastomotic stoma in their minds? Is it arterial or venous? How severe is the current bleeding? Is intervention or emergency surgery necessary? What if the condition deteriorates further? After making a preliminary judgment on abdominal hemorrhage, symptomatic treatment such as vital signs monitoring, pressor, hemostasis, blood transfusion, and fluid replacement is also required to explain the condition to the patient's family and prepare for further treatment. The above judgments and operations are to be completed in a very short time and noisy environment, in addition to the embodiment of the intervention's comprehensive medical ability and overall leadership ability, but also the test of the intervention's emotional control ability.

3.6 Keeping Pace with the Times

With the great promotion of medical field by the development of science and technology, traditional medicine has undergone dramatic changes, the cognitive field of diseases is constantly changing, and the treatment concept is also updating and changing. Intervention providers need to change, timely grasp the frontiers of discipline development, be familiar with the application methods of new therapies, new technologies, and new businesses, timely update the traditional concepts, truly keep pace with the times, and avoid following the old and stereotyped rules.

In addition to conforming to the development of medical science and technology, the times are changing, the needs of the public are changing, and medical regulations and medical environment are also changing. Intervention providers should actively cope with the changes in the new situation, continuously adjust their own intervention means, and continuously adapt to the requirements of patients and social environment for medical treatment. In addition to the disease itself, the current medical subjects should pay more attention to the sociality of the disease, emphasizing the psychological comfort to patients and the improvement of quality of life. The original surgical treatment emphasized more on the resection of the lesion and functional recovery, while now intervention providers pay attention to the satisfaction of the patient's psychological and social needs while paying attention to the therapeutic effect. For example, the traditional concept is that unresectable locally advanced pancreatic cancer can only be treated with palliative chemotherapy or radiotherapy. However, with the progress of medical concept and therapeutic drugs, many inoperable diseases can be downstaged by the induction of chemotherapy, targeted therapy, or immunotherapy, so as to obtain the chance of radical surgery, which is a subversion of the traditional treatment concept. With the development of liquid biopsy and genetic testing technology, intervention providers can also individualize the selection of targeted treatment options according to the results of tumor gene mutations, further improve the accuracy and effectiveness of treatment, so that patients can benefit from the development of science and technology. Since its inception, pancreaticoduodenectomy has been the crown jewel of abdominal surgery because of its difficulty, complicated operation steps, and high mortality rate. With the continuous improvement and refinement of the operation, the incidence of complications and mortality rate of the operation have been decreasing and the indications for the operation have been expanding. With the progress of minimally invasive surgical techniques and energy devices, laparoscopic and robotic pancreaticoduodenectomy are being applied in more and more hospitals, gradually turning giant wounds into minimally invasive, reducing the psychological burden of surgery on patients while removing the lesion and promoting the rapid recovery of patients.

3.7 Diligent in Summing Up

Advances in medicine are based on summarizing the experience of one case, finding lessons from failure, finding experiences from success, and gradually improving the intervention ability of intervention providers. Failure is a trial-and-error process, and many potential risks that cannot be seen in success can fully expose the existing problems only in failure. It is possible that the timing of treatment is not accurate, or the whole treatment plan is not comprehensive enough, if we can find the lessons learned from the failure, summarize, and make adjustments, we can completely avoid the risk and turn it into a victory. It is more important to reflect after success because success often masks many potential contradictions and risks, and if one is immersed in the joy of success without making a response, the contradictions may be concentrated. Therefore, it is necessary to find out lessons from success, find out where it is still imperfect, and take precautions in future work, so that rapid and accurate clinical decisions can be made and high-quality clinical interventions can be implemented. In the face of successful cases, it is even more necessary to summarize the lessons behind success, which cannot be masked by the joy of success, and it is necessary to consider whether there is still regret in the intervention process and whether there is the possibility of further improvement and optimization, which will become valuable experience in future interventions.

The high-risk nature of medicine lies in the potential danger of uncertainty, so surgical interventions must be done with great caution and require repeated weighing of the pros and cons in order to turn the risks into successes. However, in many cases, the intervention opportunity is fleeting, and the intervention provider must be rapid and decisive. If the intervention provider is indecisive, it often delays the timing of treatment and affects the effect of diagnosis and treatment. The self-cultivation of intervention providers lies in the ability to combine deep and solid clinical theory and practical skills, the ability to combine past courage and calm emotional control, the ability to combine multidisciplinary collaboration with doctor–patient communication ability, and the thoughtful and immediate application of clinical knowledge, experience, and technology to surgical intervention.

4 Optimization of Interventions

The uncertainty and uncontrollability of medical risks determine that medical risks are inevitable in a certain range and to a certain extent. Once the risk sources and risk factors are not effectively controlled, risk accidents and adverse consequences will still occur. Therefore, it is necessary to take active and effective measures for control and intervention, cut off the development chain of risks, and timely deal with the adverse consequences that have been caused. With the continuous development of medical science and technology, the upgrading of medical equipment, and the optimization and improvement of intervention measures and treatment options, the intervention measures have been transformed from complex to simple, to low-risk, and invasive to minimally invasive, and truly achieve the greatest benefit at the least cost. This section mainly elaborates the basic principles of intervention optimization, in order to lay a theoretical foundation for the implementation of risk control and intervention optimization.

4.1 Optimization of Intervention Means

Intervention optimization refers to the continuous improvement of interventions during clinical intervention to reduce the possible collateral damage caused by interventions and control the severity of adverse consequences to a minimum. After a risk event, all processes should be summarized and analyzed, the treatment process should be repeatedly improved, the intervention details that may increase the injury should be considered and optimized, and the risk should be faced again methodically to achieve the optimal effect with the least trauma. The implementation of interventions encompasses a process from complex to simple, from high-risk to low-risk, and invasive to minimally invasive. The process not only reflects the process of continuous understanding and in-depth understanding of diseases and pathophysiological anatomy by intervention providers, but also reflects the continuous pursuit of simple and efficient intervention measures. This is most evident in the control of bleeding in liver surgery. Hepatectomy surgery is difficult to carry out as early as possible in the absence of effective bleeding control methods, and the liver is considered to be a forbidden area for surgery. Later, the liver surgeon recognized that the hepatic blood flow into the liver was mainly provided by the hepatic artery and portal vein, and the hepatic blood flow blocking method of the first porta hepatis blocking appeared, which made hepatectomy possible. However, long-term liver ischemia will bring severe liver warm ischemia-reperfusion injury and thus lead to postoperative liver failure. It is impossible to complete difficult and large-scale hepatectomy with the first porta hepatis occlusion alone. Academician Wu Mengchao proposed the ambient temperature intermittent entry hepatic blood flow blocking technology to solve this problem well. Nowadays, with the application of minimally invasive surgery, the further understanding of liver blood flow anatomy by liver surgeons, and the accumulation of intraoperative blood control experience, doctors have continuously optimized the liver blood flow blocking technique, and a series of intraoperative bleeding control methods such as selective hemihepatic blood flow blocking method, combined lifting hemihepatic blood flow blocking method around the liver, and hepatic vein clamping blocking method to control the second porta hepatis have emerged, which greatly promote the development of liver surgery.

The measures to optimize interventions are based on three points: clinical experience, that is, continuous summary of experiences and lessons after the occurrence of risks, screening and optimization of simple and reasonable interventions in long clinical practice, and then summarizing them into theory. The summation of clinical experience does not happen overnight, but requires the induction and summary of a generation or even several generations, reflecting not only the collective wisdom of medical intervention providers, but also the "craftsmanship" that constantly pursues optimization and excellence; second, there is documentary evidence that the experience of a person or a group is limited, and the optimization and improvement that can be made is limited if it is confined to the platform and environment in which it is located alone. If we can learn advanced optimization methods for controlling risk by keeping up with the frontiers of development in our discipline with the help of current Internet informatics and smart big data, and by drawing on literature with high evidence-based medical evidence levels. Of course, the ability of intervention providers varies greatly, which is applicable to the experience and means of others and may not be well mastered by themselves. Therefore, the optimization measures still need to be organically combined with their ability in order to achieve better risk control effect; with the development of medical science and technology, science and technology are the first productivity, and the rapidly developing science and technology have brought dramatic changes to diagnostic methods, treatment means, medical equipment, etc., from the Lancet to the harmonic scalpel, Biclamp, Ligasure; from manual suture to the sealer, stapler; from laparotomy to laparoscopy to robotic surgery; from chemotherapy to targeted drugs, immunotherapy, from imaging examination to three-dimensional reconstruction, intraoperative navigation, and the development of each science and technology has brought about changes in the intervention means and treatment concept.

4.2 Implementation Principles

The optimization of intervention means is not only an improvement of single technology, but a systematic work of purpose. The following principles should be paid attention to in the implementation process:

4.2.1 Safety

The most serious consequence of medical risks for patients is the loss of life. On the basis of ensuring life safety, the goal of optimizing intervention means is to minimize the occurrence of accidental risks for patients during diagnosis and treatment and control the risks within an affordable range. With the increasing maturity of medical technology and the continuous accumulation of treatment experience, the indications for treatment are gradually relaxed, and many complex and difficult treatment means and surgical methods are implemented. However, due to the unfamiliarity and ignorance of new technologies and methods, the intervention providers cannot use them skillfully in practice, resulting in an increase in the corresponding intervention risks.

When pursuing the optimization of intervention means, intervention providers should first pay attention to ensuring the safety of medical behaviors. Surgery is a discipline with many invasive procedures and practicality. The object of operation is human. Once accidents are caused by some errors, irreversible results may be caused. Therefore, intervention providers should abide by the rules and regulations and medical principles of their specialty, strictly avoid blindly confident or afraid of assuming responsibility, and solve problems other than ability without authorization and should take ensuring safety as the first priority. Do not panic when the risk occurs, calmly evaluate, timely call a superior doctor or relevant department to assist in consultation if necessary, and effectively maintain medical safety. Medical risks often occur in some experienced intervention providers. The occurrence of risks is not due to medical technology or level problems, but due to blind self-confidence in their own ability and excessive relaxation in the diagnosis and treatment process, thus losing the ability to predict and control risks. What's more, some are even too concerned about face when the risk occurs and find it difficult to admit their own mistakes and fail to ask for help in time, thus further aggravating the damage caused by the risk.

A typical example is the grasp of indications for laparotomy during minimally invasive surgery. At present, minimally invasive surgery is the direction of surgical development, because of its small trauma and rapid recovery has become the preferred choice for doctors and patients. However, the implementation of minimally invasive surgery not only has stricter requirements for surgeons' understanding of anatomy and minimally invasive technical operation, but also has a great test for surgeons' psychology and technique for emergency treatment of a series of risks that may occur during surgery. When there is intraoperative rapid bleeding with difficulty in microscopic hemostasis; severe adhesions around the tissue, unclear anatomical levels; unplanned normal tissue damage; or when the operator's lack of skill and experience makes the operation extremely difficult, if the microscopic operation is reluctantly performed in deliberate pursuit of a lower turn-over rate, it is very likely that further medically induced injuries will occur, leading to more serious complications. Timely conversion to laparotomy is conducive to actively grasp the uncontrollable intraoperative risks, and timely treatment of side injuries that have occurred to avoid the occurrence of serious complications. We should recognize that the level of conversion rate cannot represent the technical level and proficiency of the surgeon, and conversion is not only responsible for the patient, but also a manifestation of the maturity of the surgeon, rather than a failure of the operation. An excellent minimally invasive surgeon should actively convert to laparotomy before causing serious complications and adverse consequences to patients according to the specific intraoperative circumstances and the experience and technical level of the surgeon. All invasive operations should be based on the premise of ensuring the safety of patients.

4.2.2 Effectiveness

After the first goal of ensuring the life safety of patients, intervention providers should also consider how to obtain the greatest risk control effect at the least cost, which requires continuous balance among risks, benefits, and costs and screening the most economical and reasonable combination of intervention means and options.

By effectiveness, we mean that the cost is reasonable, unnecessary expenses are minimized, and the cost of risk control measures is kept as low as possible. Objectively speaking, cost reduction often affects the ultimate effectiveness of risk prevention, so balancing cost and benefit become the key to achieving this goal. The balance between cost (economic and human cost of risk control) and benefit (degree of patient benefit and safety) needs to be weighed on a practical basis. Any risk prevention measures are costly, and the control measures taken and the protection of the patient should be adapted to the severity of the consequences that may be caused. If excessive prevention of low-risk accidents easily costs too much effort, the high-risk factors that really need to be taken should be ignored.

Clinically, whether patients after surgery need to be monitored in the ICU and the length of time involves the problem of effectiveness. If some patients are not admitted to ICU, they cannot be closely and meticulously monitored after operation, and the risk of postoperative complications is difficult to be well monitored and prevented. If the monitoring time in ICU is too long, it will cause hospitalization costs, and the treatment of professional diseases may affect the final recovery of patients due to the lack of monitoring by specialist medical staff. Therefore, the pursuit of benefit maximization in the medical process is also the process to achieve the optimization of intervention means, and individualized intervention programs need to be formed through continuous practice and repeated optimization in the clinical process.

4.2.3 Cooperativity

The process of therapeutic intervention is actually the process of internal communication in medical institutions, mutual cooperation between intervention providers, and strengthening cooperation. In the traditional diagnosis and treatment process, we pay more attention to the patient's condition and the implementation of management measures, and it is very easy to ignore the importance of internal communication among intervention providers. In dealing with medical risks, intervention providers often care more about their own concerned and familiar areas and problems, but ignore the overall planning. The integrity of medicine determines that it is necessary to strengthen the internal cooperation of medical treatment. The purpose of controlling risks can be achieved through the cooperation of many intervention providers. First of all, medical management personnel should establish an education system for risk pre-control, provide knowledge and background education on risk prevention and control to front-line medical care, so that they understand the principles and methods of risk prevention and control. At the same time, clinical intervention providers, including doctors, nurses, and caregivers, should have a collective awareness and the concept of mutual cooperation. In clinical work, because the serious consequences caused by unclear explanation of the condition and weak risk awareness are common when handing over with the shift, the physician on duty, and the nurse on duty, this requires the intervention providers at all levels to do a good job in risk exchange, hand over the relay baton to control medical risks, and ensure the safety of patients. In addition, it is emphasized that comprehensive and detailed risk exchange can be carried out among multiple disciplines, and through communication and discussion of related disciplines, the advantages are complementary to achieve the best comprehensive diagnosis, treatment, and risk control effect.

When a patient requires complex surgery, it is time to test the ability of the team to collaborate with each other. The author has treated a patient with pancreatic cancer who underwent 3 stents for coronary stenosis. The patient required pancreaticoduodenectomy as soon as possible due to tumor development. However, the patient had been at surgical risk for coronary stent implantation for just more than a month. The patient's multiple organ function was greatly tested after surgery, and signs of heart failure, respiratory failure, and renal failure occurred at one time. Through repeated consultation and communication in the Department of Cardiology, the Department of Respiratory Medicine, and the Department of Nephrology, as well as close monitoring by ICU medical staff, the patient finally turned to safety with the full cooperation of various physicians and nurses, reflecting the importance and necessity of cooperation and cooperation between multidisciplinary and various intervention providers.

4.2.4 Controllability

Prognosis control surgical theory contains the concept of active coping and active intervention, fully reflecting the ability of intervention providers to understand and treat the disease. The intervention means need to be operable, through the optimization and simplification of the operation process, to form a standardized control program that is easy to implement and promote. Although risk control varies from person to person, and different intervention providers have different risk understanding and control abilities, the ultimate purpose of medical treatment is to benefit patients. In order to allow more patients to obtain better therapeutic effect and avoid or reduce the risks caused by the disease itself and therapeutic operation, we must repeatedly optimize the intervention program and improve its ease of operation.

One scholar once said that if only one of a certain technology or operation mode is completed, even if this technology or operation mode is no higher level and no more advanced, it has no value of existence and promotion. The existence value of a disease intervention technology or means lies not only in that it can solve a difficult problem to conquer in clinical practice, but also in whether it can be popularized on a large scale to benefit more patients and even promote the progress of a treatment plan or concept. The author's proposed laparoscopic patterned left lateral lobectomy is such a technical system. In the past, laparoscopic resection of the left lateral lobe of the liver was not a simple surgical procedure, and laparoscopic hepatectomy bleeding was difficult to control due to the dual blood supply system of the liver and hepatic venous return system, which was not easy for even experienced liver surgeons to master. Through the systematic study on the vascular anatomy of the left lateral lobe of the liver and the repeated screening of hepatectomy tools, we propose that laparoscopic patterned left lateral lobectomy of the liver can quickly transect the liver without the need for additional blood flow occlusion through a simple and easy two-step method, which not only allows more liver surgeons to complete this, but also allows more patients to obtain the rapid rehabilitation experience brought about by minimally invasive treatment and accelerates the minimally invasive process of liver surgery.

4.3 Significance

In the past, we mainly coped with medical risks based on passive coping and lacked awareness of active intervention. Today, we should do a good job in risk control, enhance the early warning awareness of intervention providers for disease risks and intervention risks, improve risk identification and evaluation ability, change the uncontrollable risks into controllable through continuous optimization of intervention measures, and simplify and regularize the operation of complex risks. Only by running the concept of risk control and optimization of intervention means throughout the medical process, considering the hidden dangers of treatment as the risks to be controlled, is the practical application of the idea of prevention-oriented and control optimization. Through the continuous optimization of specific measures of intervention means, it is conducive to overcoming the passive and blind risk treatment methods in the traditional treatment methods, reducing medical risks, and promoting the overall progress of medical technology and concepts.

The role of applying the optimization theory of interventions in the medical field is mainly reflected in the following four aspects:

1. Doing intervention risk front-loading: Risk control is not just a matter of doing things, but of doing things in advance to control risk. Through a large number of experience summarization in clinical practice, the implementation of intervention before the occurrence of risks to achieve advanced control can effectively prevent the passivity and loss of control when the risks occur and minimize the hazards caused by risks.
2. Revealing the root cause of the problem: The fundamental point of risk control lies in grasping the crux of the problem through the risk appearance, exploring the causes and root causes of medical risks, continuously optimizing the intervention means according to the pathophysiological characteristics of different diseases and the principle of treatment operation, and taking control measures from the source, rather than grasping the details of the problem.
3. Fine risk management: Risk control not only emphasizes independent and single risk control methods, but also systematically recognizes and solves the risk problems existing in the diagnosis and treatment of diseases and realizes fine and optimized risk management through the continuous optimization of intervention means and refining them into the various elements of disease laws and anatomical characteristics.
4. Effective doctor–patient communication: Due to the complete asymmetry of information between doctors and patients in terms of medical knowledge, the occurrence of medical risks is often the fuse that triggers medical dispute accidents. Therefore, through the optimization of active and effective intervention means, the therapeutic effect of patients can be improved, the prognosis can be improved, and it is conducive to the establishment of a harmonious and good medical environment and doctor–patient relationship.

5 Selection of Intervention Timing

Can we obtain the best prognostic effect if we master the first three elements in the process of clinical diagnosis and treatment mentioned above? The answer is certainly no, because we neglect one of the most critical factors, and this factor is the lubricant that combines intervention providers, means of intervention, and disease risk. As the saying goes, everything is ready but the east wind and the factor we are going to talk about here is the so-called east wind, that is, the intervention timing. The intervention timing we emphasize is not only important in the field of life and death medicine, but also in the long history of military struggles and business games, where the timing is crucial. Good disease risk control can only be obtained with the right interventions at the right time, while if the intervention is at the wrong time, it is difficult to obtain good outcomes even with a focused team of intervention providers and the most advanced interventions.

5.1 Selection of Intervention Timing

The so-called intervention timing is the time node for intervention providers to apply interventions to control and intervene in disease risk. Popularly speaking, it is the time and cycle of treatment, and in clinical practice intervention providers need to make a large number of choices about the intervention timing every day. The choice of intervention timing is not only affected by disease risk, intervention provider, and intervention means, but also can act backwards on disease risk and affect the effect of intervention and the prognosis of patients.

Of course, the intervention timing is not static. When the risk of disease and the corresponding intervention providers and intervention means change, the selection of intervention timing should also be adjusted accordingly, that is, the dynamic optimization of intervention timing. Dynamic optimization of intervention timing requires intervention providers to be able to flexibly grasp the intervention timing and be the overall manager of clinical intervention, rather than rigid and rigid executors, and intervention providers are good at thinking, comprehensively grasp various elements of prognosis control medicine, and carry out reasonable allocation and optimal combination.

5.2 Classification

We divided the other three factors into three categories according to their effects on the intervention timing, that is, the timing related to disease risk, the timing related to intervention providers, and the timing related to intervention means, which together constitute the crucial impact of the intervention timing on the prognosis of patients.

5.2.1 Timing Related to Disease Risk

The intervention timing must be adapted to the risk of the disease, because the intervention goal of prognosis control medicine is the control of the disease, and the risk of the disease is also the main body of the intervention, so what kind of disease risk determines when the intervention needs to be performed. Surgery can be divided into emergency surgery, limited surgery, and elective surgery, the difference between the three lies in the intervention timing. Emergency surgery requires intervention in the first place, which requires every minute, and if delayed, the best time for intervention will be fleeting, resulting in irreversible losses. Limited surgery is not so demanding on the timeliness of intervention and can be flexibly mastered within a certain range, of course, the time node cannot be delayed without restriction, so as not to cause disease progression or deterioration. Elective surgery often appears in the treatment of benign diseases, because its disease risk is the lowest, the impact on patients is small, so the timeliness of the intervention is required, and it can be performed electively. The above differences in the intervention timing are closely related to the criticality and severity of disease risk, and intervention providers need to reasonably select the intervention timing according to the priority of disease risk. Only when the intervention is performed at a reasonable time, the clinical thinking of the intervention provider can be fully combined with the optimized intervention to control the disease risk within a minimum range.

5.2.2 Timing Related to Intervention Providers

The intervention provider is the determiner of the intervention timing and the implementer of the means of the intervention and plays a leading role throughout the control of disease risk and the intervention process. When is the best timing for intervention? The answer to this question does not come out of thin air and is not static, requiring intervention providers to use their subjective initiative to continuously optimize the intervention timing in repeated experience accumulation and clinical evidence update and come from practice to practice, so as to maximize the benefits of intervention. Conversely, humans are also their emotional animals, susceptible to external and internal factors, in their poor emotional state if reluctantly implemented intervention may affect the effect of treatment, and even threaten the patient's life. Risk control of diseases is a major event related to the safety of life and must not affect the treatment of diseases due to emotional factors, so when the intervention provider is emotionally disturbed, it is necessary to adjust the intervention timing or replace the intervention provider according to the situation. For example, if a surgeon has uncontrollable mood swings before surgery due to family or work reasons, if the surgery is performed reluctantly, it may affect the operator's observation, judgment, resilience, and concentration during the surgery, which will eventually affect the outcome of the surgery and the patient's recovery, or even worse, may cause irreversible consequences due to mistakes, the best choice is to ask a senior or fellow surgeon to replace the surgeon if it is an emergency surgery, or to change the operation time to avoid unnecessary intervention risks if it is an elective surgery.

5.2.3 Timing Related to Intervention Means

In the past decade, medical science and technology have developed extremely rapidly, bringing about a change from diagnosis to treatment, from drugs to devices. With the development and change of diagnosis and treatment experience and treatment concept, it brings not only the optimization and upgrading of intervention means, but also the change of relevant timing of intervention means to medicine. In other words, traditional interventions do not seize the best intervention timing, and with the continuous update of interventions can achieve the continuous optimization of the intervention timing. For example, in the treatment of congenital heart disease in infants and young children, since the traditional extracorporeal circulation technique will induce the release of a large number of inflammatory factors in the body, resulting in increased vascular permeability, resulting in severe tissue edema and cardiopulmonary dysfunction in children, and even leading to the death of children, the previous concept mostly recommends surgical treatment after the children reach adulthood. However, the disease will continue to progress during this time, and if the condition deteriorates further, the child may not be able to undergo surgery. In addition, while waiting for surgery, the child will suffer from the disease and lose the opportunity to enjoy a good childhood as a healthy child. At present, with the application of ultrafiltration technology in cardiac surgery with cardiopulmonary bypass in children, it can significantly reduce intraoperative blood loss and blood transfusion volume, improve pulmonary oxygenation function, improve postoperative cardiopulmonary function, so that once the disease in children is found, there is an opportunity to perform radical surgery. The acquisition of this intervention timing is inseparable from the development of science and technology and the progress of intervention means.

5.3 How to Grasp the Intervention Timing

The intervention timing we talked before is often based on the experience of intervention providers or the basis of evidence-based medicine, however, it is impossible to have exactly the same disease and exactly the same patient, so it is impossible to completely learn from the previous experience or the concept of others. If we can summarize how to grasp the best time to intervene in the treatment from a scientific and quantitative perspective, we will be able to learn from the past and make full use of the maximum effectiveness of the intervener and the intervention tools in the future intervention process. We talk about the best intervention timing, that is, according to the change of intervention benefits and intervention risks, select the timing with the greatest difference between the two. In practical clinical work, the selection of intervention timing should follow the following decision sequence: ①: judge whether the intervention risk is lower than the intervention benefit, and the timing of intervention risk is higher than the intervention benefit cannot implement the intervention; ②: judge whether the intervention benefit and intervention risk will change when meeting ①, if the difference between the expected intervention benefit and the intervention risk will increase, select to wait, otherwise select to intervene as early as possible; ③: when failing to meet ①, seek the auxiliary intervention means that can reduce the intervention risk or improve the intervention benefit, optimize the intervention means, if still unable to meet ①, change the intervention goal and the combination of intervention provider/intervention means for re-evaluation, and stop the intervention when unable to meet ① under realistic conditions.

5.3.1 Safety

The core of medical treatment lies in safety, and the choice of intervention timing is the same. Ensuring the patient's life and health is the first goal to determine the intervention timing. With the continuous progress of intervention means and the continuous improvement of technical experience, the indications for treatment are gradually relaxed, which includes not only more and more opportunities for the treatment of intractable diseases, but also more and more extensive requirements for the intervention timing. For example, if acute cholecystitis has occurred for more than 48 h in the past, conservative treatment is recommended to prevent organ and duct injury caused by tissue inflammation and edema. With the development of laparoscopic techniques and the accumulation of surgeon experience, many patients can also perform minimally invasive surgery in the inflammatory phase and obtain a good therapeutic effect. However, with the consequent accidental injury of hepatic artery and bile duct, some of them will even bring irreversible injury and pain to patients and even threaten the life safety of patients. Therefore, the author does not advocate violating medical principles to relieve the limitation of the intervention timing and even broadening the indications for treatment for the benefit of patients should be based on adequate preparation and improvement of their own ability.

5.3.2 Efficacy

After ensuring patient safety, the intervention provider should consider how to continuously balance the risks and benefits of the intervention, and the best timing for intervention is when judging the maximum difference between the benefits and risks of the intervention. The pursuit of maximizing the benefit of patients is also a process of continuously adjusting the intervention timing, which needs to be achieved by intervention providers through continuous practice and repeated optimization in the clinical process, closely following the forefront of medical science and technology development. Of course, with the development of medicine, the optimal intervention timing is relative, and as long as the intervention timing can benefit patients clinically is an effective intervention timing. The intervention timing is actually a cross-sectional area. In this cross-sectional area, the intervention provider, intervention means, and disease risks are certain, and the intervention benefits and intervention risks brought about are also certain. What the intervention provider has to do is to ensure that the risk–benefit difference can achieve the ultimate goal of benefiting the patients in each cross-sectional area where the intervention is implemented. For example, for intraductal papillary mucinous tumors of the pancreas, surgical resection is the only effective treatment. However, when the tumor diameter is <3 cm, the probability of malignant transformation of the tumor is very low, and the risk of pancreatic surgery is greater. The expected benefit of intervention is significantly lower than the risk of intervention. At this time, the selection of surgical treatment is not the best time, but follow-up observation should be selected. However, when the tumor growth rate is fast, or the tumor diameter exceeds 3 cm, it is considered that the possibility of malignant transformation of the tumor is high. At this time, the rapidly increasing risk of disease has significantly exceeded the risk of intervention for surgery, so immediate surgical treatment is required.

5.3.3 Dynamics

The so-called optimal intervention timing is actually relative, rather than absolute. The intervention timing for the same disease is also different, and decisions need to be made dynamically according to the degree of development and risk changes of the disease. For example, for the same acute calculous cholecystitis, emergency cholecystectomy should be performed within 48 h after the onset of the disease to remove the lesion most quickly and effectively. When the onset of cholecystitis exceeds 48 h, the inflammation and edema of the gallbladder and surrounding tissues are severe. If reluctant surgical treatment is easy to cause serious complications such as bile duct and vascular injury, if such conditions are encountered, the patient should be advised to perform conservative treatment for 3 months. The inflammation and edema of the gallbladder and surrounding tissues are reduced. After the risk of intervention is reduced, this is the best timing for intervention and intervention can be performed. However, the dynamic development and uncertainty of the disease may lead to secondary acute obstructive suppurative cholangitis. This disease is more dangerous and can lead to systemic inflammatory response syndrome, induce multiple organ failure and even patient death. At this time, emergency surgical treatment is required after weighing the advantages and disadvantages. Therefore, the dynamic nature of the disease risk determines the dynamic nature of the intervention timing and needs to view the problem with the perspective of dynamic development.

5.4 Significance

The intervention timing is an "invisible and untouchable" subjective factor in the medical process, which does not exist in isolation, but is interconnected and interacts with disease risk, intervention providers, and intervention means, which together constitute the four elements of prognosis control medicine. It is very important to select the best intervention time according to the disease risk, the interrelationship between intervention providers and intervention means to maximize the benefits of patients, which has realistic guiding significance for clinical work. On the one hand, reasonable intervention timing can enable the intervention provider to exert the greatest subjective initiative, make full use of their clinical thinking and optimized intervention means to better make decisions and implement interventions, on the other hand, reasonable intervention timing can also jump out of the limitations and confinements of medical level and platform to the intervention provider and intervention means, so that the patients can obtain the best treatment results within the existing diagnosis and treatment level and intervention ability range.

Suggested Reading

Askren A, Leslie P. Complexity of clinical decision making: consent, capacity, and ethics. Semin Speech Lang. 2019;40(3):162–9.

Bartoli FG, Arnone GB, Ravera G, et al. Pancreatic fistula and relative mortality in malignant disease after pancreaticoduodenectomy. Review and statistical meta-analysis regarding 15 years of literature. Anticancer Res. 1991;11(11):1831–48.

Chen GT, Liu ZM. Theory and practice of damage control surgery. J Surg Concepts Pract. 2005;10(2):197–8.

Donati M, Stavrou GA, Donati A, et al. The risk of spontaneous rupture of liver hemangiomas: a critical review of the literature. J Hepatobiliary Pancreat Sci. 2011;18(6):797.

Evidence-Based Medicine Working Group. Evidence-based medicine. A new approach to teaching the practice of medicine. JAMA. 1992;268(17):2420–5.

Gamborg ML, Mehlsen M, Paltved C, et al. Conceptualizations of clinical decision-making: a scoping review in geriatric emergency medicine. BMC Emerg Med. 2020;20(1):73.

Gary H. McCullough, Balaji Rangarathnam. Clinical Decision Making. Semin Speech Lang. 2019;40(3):149–50.

Giuliante F, Ardito F, Vellone M, et al. Reappraisal of surgical indications and approach for liver hemangioma: single-center experience on 74 patients. Am J Surg. 2011;201(6):741–8.

Greenhalgh T, Howick J, Maskrey N, Evidence Based Medicine Renaissance Group. Evidence based medicine: a movement in crisis? BMJ. 2014;48:3725.

Han QD. Improving the humanistic quality of doctors. Orthop J Chin. 2007;21:2100.

Hoekstra LT, Bieze M, Erdogan D, et al. Management of giant liver hemangiomas: an update. Expert Rev Gastroenterol Hepatol. 2013;7(3):263–8.

Hoopes CW, Kukreja J, Golden J, et al. Extracorporeal membrane oxygenation as a bridge to pulmonary transplantation. J Thorac Cardiovasc Surg. 2013;145(3):862–7.

Huang ZQ. Strive to improve the therapeutic effect on severe acute cholangitis. Chin J Pract Surg. 1986;6:12.

Kozlowski D, Hutchinson M, Hurley J, et al. The role of emotion in clinical decision making: an integrative literature review. BMC Med Educ. 2017;17(1):255.

Li JS. Improving the quality of adhesive small bowel obstruction surgery. Chin J Pract Surg. 2000;8:4–6.

Li HY, Liang B, Li RZ. The unification of modern medical science and humanistic spirit and the cultivation of comprehensive quality of clinicians. Med Philos. 2004;25(8):32–3.

Liu R. Medical intervention should focus on prognosis - dynamic prognosis control in medicine. Acad J Chin PLA Med School. 2018;39(11):1–3.

Liu R, Hu MG. Discussion on several problems of laparoscopic anatomical hepatectomy: 10-year experience of Chinese PLA General Hospital. Chin J Surg. 2010;3(6):466–73.

Liu Q, Liu R. Intraoperative risk control and minimally invasive Hepatopancreatobiliary surgery. Chin J Laparosc Surg. 2017;10(2):65–8.

Lowy AM, Lee JE, Pisters PW, et al. Prospective, randomized trial of octreotide to prevent pancreatic fistula after pancreaticoduodenectomy for malignant disease. Ann Surg. 1997;226(5):632.

Mao WJ, Chen JY. Application of extracorporeal membrane oxygenation in pretransplant support transition. Chin J Organ Transplant. 2011;2(4):209–16.

Qiao HQ, Jiang HC. Talking about the cultivation of surgeon quality. Chin J Pract Surg. 2004;24(1):9–11.

Qin SH. Physicians, medical arts and humanities. Tsinghua University Press; 2007.

Rungsakulkij N, Mingphruedhi S, Tangtawee P, et al. Risk factors for pancreatic fistula following pancreaticoduodenectomy: a retrospective study in a Thai tertiary center. World J Gastrointest Surg. 2017;9(12):270–80.

Sara JDS, Toya T, Rihal CS, et al. Clinical decision-making: challenging traditional assumptions. Int J Cardiol. 2021;326:6–11.

Schnelldorfer T, Ware AL, Smoot R, et al. Management of giant hemangioma of the liver: resection versus observation. J Am Coll Surg. 2010;211(6):724–30.

Shi LP, Huang SH, Zheng ZH, Liu JR, Su YB. Timing analysis of operation for acute severe cholecystitis. Chin J Gen Surg. 2018;27(2):225–30.

Tian YH, Xu Z, Zhang XQ. Discussion on the cultivation of humanistic quality of surgeons. Med Philos. 2010;31(2):69–71.

Tranvåg EJ, Norheim OF, Ottersen T. Clinical decision making in cancer care: a review of current and future roles of patient age. BMC Cancer. 2018;18(1):546.

Wang F, Liu R. Intelligent surgery: changing trends in surgical practice patterns. Acad J Second Milit Med Univ. 2018;39(8):830–3.
Yan XY, Dong CY, Yao C. Evidence-based medicine research in the era of big data. Chin J Evid Based Med. 2017;17(3):249–54.
Yang WB, Meng QM. Application of cost-benefit analysis in hospital economic management. Econ Res Guide. 2018;16:110–1.
Zhao GD, Hu MG, Liu R. Patterned laparoscopic left lateral lobectomy: a report of 71 cases. J Southern Med Univ. 2011;4:737–40.

Surgical Risk Management

2

Rong Liu, Hongchen Ji, and Ruiquan Zhou

Abstract

This chapter begins with a brief review of the development of surgery and surgical risks in different periods. Then the surgical risk pre-control system is introduced in detail, which can be divided into risk identification, assessment and prevention, and risk control according to whether the risk occurs. In the section on surgical risk identification, a variety of common surgical risks and methods for risk identification are described. In the section of surgical risk assessment, common surgical risk assessment methods and common predictive scoring models are introduced. In the section of risk intervention, the principles of risk intervention and the two major forms of intervention, risk prevention and risk control, are described.

1 Definition of Surgical Risk

Surgery is an important part of medical science and one of the main branches of clinical medicine. Surgery, from the Latin "Chirurgia," evolved from a combination of Greek "Cheir" (hand) and "Ergon" (work), implying that surgery is a discipline closely related to operation.

The concept, category, therapeutic means and tools of surgery, as well as the medical problems that can be solved, gradually change with the progress of human history. Especially in the past two centuries, the wave brought about by the industrial revolution and the explosion of science and technology has led to the rapid development of surgery. Today, the establishment of the surgical giant tower is inseparable from the exploration and discovery of predecessors, efforts to innovate

R. Liu (✉) · H. Ji · R. Zhou
Faculty of Hepato-pancreato-biliary Surgery, Chinese PLA General Hospital, Beijing, China
e-mail: liurong301@127.com

R. Liu (ed.), *Clinical Decision Making for Improving Prognosis*,
https://doi.org/10.1007/978-981-19-2952-6_2

and experience summary; as contemporary medical workers, we should also pay tribute to all patients and their families who provide help for the development of surgery and even the entire medical cause. However, it is undeniable that the development of surgery has been a thorny path of innovation and risk, and a brief review of the history of the development of surgery will help to recognize the surgical risks that have occurred, resolved, and unresolved, throughout history.

1.1 Ancient Surgery

1.1.1 The Origin of Surgery

Surgery has an early origin as the basic treatment, and according to archeological findings, the ancient Inca of South America in 3000 BC have been able to perform initial craniotomies. Craniotomies in Inca are not only used as a treatment, but also contain components of witchcraft. However, it remains unclear what kind of anesthesia, hemostasis, and anti-infection techniques was used by the Incas to get the patient through the operation and survive long term.

Until 1600 BC, the first surgical work in human history, the Edwin Smith Papyrus in ancient Egypt, was completed. It can be considered the earliest medical literature on neurosurgery with the application of a standardized case record approach to 48 common accidental traumas and containing craniotomies to reduce intracranial pressure. In addition, the diagnosis and treatment of spinal injury, chin dislocation, various fractures, and so on have also been very accurately recorded.

1.1.2 Hippocrates and Galen

By the fifth century BC–the fourth century BC, the Hippocratic Oath by Hippocrates (460–370 B.C.), the "father of medicine," included a passage that read, "Nor will I give a woman a pessary to produce abortion…I will not cut for stone, even for patients in whom the disease is manifest; I will leave this operation to be performed by practitioners, specialists in this art." It recognizes the skill of surgeons, distinguishes surgery from internal medicine, and has had a profound impact in the history of Western medicine. However, the negative impact of this oath also perpetuated the view of surgery as a dirty, low-level medicine for a long time, due to the small scope of surgical applications, the high degree of injury and the high risks involved.

Galen (Galen, 129–216 A.D.) living in ancient Rome is another surgical giant in the history of medicine. He conducted numerous studies of human anatomy and boldly performed unprecedented brain and eye surgeries and is said to be co-authored more than 500 works. But as Galen's writings spread, they gradually degenerated into dogma, forming "Galenism." Galen's "five-lobe theory of the liver" and bloodletting therapy have been fetishized by later generations: the former (note: different from the anatomical segment of the eight segments of the five lobes of the liver today) was still embraced by university professors at the time until 1500 years later and was considered "variant" even in the face of the liver in the dissected corpse; the latter had a more profound impact, even to the end of the eighteenth century, the U.S. Founding Father George Washington (1732–1799 A.D.)

suffered from an acute upper respiratory tract infection causing respiratory obstruction, the physician at the time used bloodletting instead of tracheotomy, which not only did not work but caused hemorrhagic shock, Washington died that night.

The doctrines of Hippocrates and Galen have had a profound influence on later generations: physicians in medieval Europe generally believed that contaminating blood damaged their dignity, while churches, which held great power at the time, did not regard surgery as an important medicine, but only as a last resort, and the absence of anesthesia at that time made the reputation of surgeons poor; in addition, if the treatment results were poor, the personal safety of surgeons would even be threatened. As a result, the status of surgeons at that time was low and most of them also worked as barbers, and the guilds of barber-surgeons were established in England in 1540. According to legend, the red, blue, and white barrels rotating in front of modern hair salons represent arteries, veins, and bandages. It was not until after the Renaissance that anatomy was intensively studied and combined with surgery, and surgery was truly separated from the category of the manual industry.

The origin of surgery in China is very early. In the Zhou Dynasty, there was a setting of medical administration and a division of medical treatment, and the surgeons were called "royal surgeons." Zhou Li Tianguan recorded that their responsibilities were: "royal surgeons are responsible for treating abscess, ulcer, open incised wound and fracture." "The Master of surgery" Hua Tuo (145–208 B.C) used "anesthesia powder" for anesthesia and "scraping the bones to heal the wound," which left a heavy mark in the history of surgical development in China. However, due to the lack of exploration of anatomy, surgery has not taken root and thrived in China.

Although ancient surgery also has a shining moment, it is generally limited by the development restrictions of basic science, religious politics, and the ideological shackles of feudal superstition, and the development is very slow. At the same time, surgery has a very high risk, pain, bleeding, infection and other surgical risks are "unbearable pain." How to solve this series of surgical risks is the main theme of the next development of surgery.

1.2 Modern Surgery

The core issues surrounding the entire history of surgery—pain, infection, and bleeding—are surgical risks that have always plagued surgeons. The fact that the patient is in great pain and in extreme shock during surgery has forced surgery in the direction of speed and has even created a wave of racing among surgeons. The most famous of them is Robert Liston (1794–1847 A.D.), a British doctor who is said to be able to complete amputation of one leg in 29 s, and amputation and suturing of one arm within 90 s. What is even more "famous" is that he completed a thriller surgery with a mortality rate of 300%: in an amputation, Liston quickly sawed the injured thigh and accidentally cut the finger of the assistant holding the injured on the side, and both the patient and the assistant died of postoperative infection; and the third death was in the audience watching the operation on the side, who died of shock due to the bloody and horrible surgical process.

Although this unique surgery with 300% mortality seems absurd, it is a true portrayal in the era of lack of effective anesthesia and anti-infective means. Dr. Liston, however, is not a so-called quack, but a very famous surgeon at that time, which suggests that good prognosis cannot be absolutely achieved for patients through personal superb medical skills alone, and we need various advanced technical support from the development of basic disciplines to reduce surgical risks.

1.2.1 Establishment and Application of Anesthesia

It was not until the nineteenth century that physicians used inhalational anesthetics for surgical anesthesia to solve the problem of intraoperative pain. It is now generally accepted that the first use of ether as an anesthetic was by Crawford Long (1815–1878 A.D.), an American country surgeon, who used ether inhalation anesthesia to remove a 1.5-inch tumor from the back of the neck of a patient on March 30, 1842, and the patient did not feel pain. But because of his remote location, his achievements were known to colleagues and friends at the time and were not reported until 1848. Another founder of surgical anesthesia was Horace Wells (1815–1848 A.D.), an American dentist who was inspired by a tour of laughing gas and used laughing gas as an anesthetic on himself in 1844, allowing the assistant to extract a wisdom tooth without pain. In 1845, Wells did a public performance at the Massachusetts General Hospital in Boston with the help of his student William T.G. Morton (1819–1868 A.D), but the amount of anesthetic was insufficient and the patient shouted for pain, so Wells was driven out of the door and his reputation was greatly affected. Inspired by Wells, on October 16, 1846, Morton was recommended by his friends to come to the operating room of Massachusetts General Hospital and publicly performed test surgery under ether anesthesia, and he extracted the patient's teeth with the patient almost unconscious. Since this anesthesia has been promoted around the world, intraoperative pain is no longer a difficult problem for surgeons.

1.2.2 Surgical Disinfection and Antibiotics

The theoretical basis of surgical disinfection methods mainly comes from the experiment of gooseneck flasks by the French microbiologist Louis Pasteur (1822–1895) in the 1860s. Pasteur filled the broth into the common flask and the gooseneck flask, respectively, with the opening of the flask and the external air in contact with the broth surface, and finally the broth in the gooseneck flask did not spoil. By clever design, their findings confirmed that bacteria were responsible for the spoilage of substances.

British surgeon Joseph Lister (1827–1912) was deeply inspired to start studying the problem of anti-infection in surgery and first proposed that lack of disinfection is the main cause of infection after surgery. Lister believes that the best way to prevent postoperative infection is to eliminate bacteria before they enter the exposed wound. Lister used carbol phenol as a sterilizing agent and asked the doctor to wash his hands before surgery and establish a new sterilization method using disinfected instruments and gauze. In 1867, Lister summarized and published the research results on sterilization; after a long period of preaching and demonstration experiments, his sterilization principle was finally widely accepted by the medical community, and Lister was also known as the "father of surgical disinfection."

By 1929, the British microbiologist Alexander Fleming (1881–1955) discovered penicillin and was mass-produced at the end of World War II, thus rapidly reversing the allied war. After the war, penicillin was more widely used, saving tens of millions of lives. Since then, a series of antibiotics have been discovered and synthesized, and the problem of surgical infection has been greatly solved.

1.2.3 Hemostatic Techniques and Blood Transfusion

In the sixteenth century, medical development made people realize that disinfection should be performed for gunshot wounds and other war wounds to prevent infection, but at that time, the regular authoritative disinfection and hemostasis method was very cruel—the use of boiling oil or burning red iron for high temperature disinfection of the wound and cauterization of arterial hemostasis, which brought great pain to patients. The famous medical scientist Ambroise Paré (1501–1590 A.D.) advocated cleaning and treating the wound. It is reported that he used up the boiling oil when treating the wounded at one time. Rose oil, egg yolk, and turpentine were mixed into mixed ointment and applied to the wound to reduce the pain. For the first time, vascular ligation and hemostasis were applied to the wound for hemostasis, and it was applied and popularized. Paré's contribution has made a significant change in traditional surgery and also improved the status of surgeons to some extent, and the medical community agrees that he is the "father of modern surgery."

The development of hemostatic technology not only benefits from the proficiency of surgeons in operating skills, but also relies on the invention and improvement of hemostatic devices. In 1871, Spencer Wells (1818–1897 A.D.), a famous British surgeon, improved on the basis of the hemostatic forceps invented by predecessors and designed three to four positioning teeth, greatly improving the hemostatic effect. In 1873, the German surgeon Friedrich von Esmarch (1823-1908 A.D.) invented the tourniquet—the application of a strong flat rubber bandage, which first expels blood flow from the limb by gravity or compression, and then encircles the limb to block circulation.

In 1901, Landsteiner discovered the blood type and won the Nobel Prize in Medicine in 1930. The first person to use Landsteiner's blood group theory to guide clinical transfusions was Carrel, who had successfully connected the artery of the transfused person to the vein of the recipient in 1906 and since then blood transfusion can be used to compensate for blood loss during surgery. At the early stage, the direct blood transfusion method was used, but the operation was complex and the blood transfusion volume was not easy to control; in 1915, Lewisohn in Germany proposed the indirect blood transfusion method in which the blood was not coagulated by the mixed sodium rafter solution, and then the establishment of blood bank made the blood transfusion simple and easy.

Blood transfusion is an important method to save patients with excessive blood loss, and the first blood transfusion experiment in the history of medicine was performed by the French physician Jean-Baptiste Denys (1643–1704 A.D). On June 15, 1667, he transfused a boy and a middle-aged man successively by connecting a lamb artery to a human vein with a silver tube, and two patients eventually survived. However, direct transfusion of animal blood into humans would result in severe hemolytic reactions, and several patients in subsequent experiments were in serious danger or even died, and this method of transfusion was quickly condemned and banned. Until the early nineteenth century, the British physician Brendley envisaged saving the lives of patients with postpartum hemorrhage with blood transfusion therapy and designed a set of blood transfusion equipment for blood transfusion, resulting in 5 of 10 patients obtained benefits. In the Franco-Prussian War between 1870 and 1871, blood transfusion was largely used to save injured soldiers.

In 1900, when the Austrian pathologist Karl Landsteiner (1968–1943 A.D.) worked at the Institute of Pathology in Vienna, he found that one person's serum sometimes agglutinated with another person's red blood cells. Subsequently, Landsteiner performed cross-mixing experiments with normal blood from 22 colleagues and found that human blood could be divided into different types according to different antigens and antibodies in red blood cells and serum, and he represented the three different types of blood he found with three letters: A, B, and O. In 1902, Landsteiner's students expanded their experimental awareness to 155 people and further discovered blood type AB. In 1927, the original alphabetic nomenclature of Landsteiner was officially adopted internationally, which identified the four blood groups A, B, O, and AB. So far, the modern blood group system has been officially established. Later, with the invention of the method of preserving blood with sodium citrate solution and the introduction of the concept of blood component transfusion, blood transfusion technology has become more and more mature.

After world history entered the modern era, the waves of the Renaissance and the Industrial Revolution gave a strong boost to the development of medicine, and surgical risks such as intraoperative pain, surgical infection, and intraoperative hemostasis, which were previously insurmountable due to the technological limitations of the times, were largely solved in this era.

1.3 Modern Surgery

Prior to the nineteenth century, surgery often left an impression of bloody operations and terrible complications and mortality. By the twentieth century, several major problems that plague surgery have been basically solved; while the two World Wars have brought great pain to mankind, their strong stimulation of politics, economy, and science has laid the foundation for the rapid development of surgery. Thanks to the technological advances of the last half century, surgical aids have been completely revolutionized, and surgical procedures are pursued with greater refinement and minimal invasiveness. Surgery in the new era is no longer a manual technique, but a comprehensive discipline based on anatomy, physiology, pathology, experimental science and evidence-based medicine, synthesizing ethics and psychology, and promoting the progress of surgical techniques towards higher levels.

1.3.1 Standardization and Specialization of Surgery

Into the twentieth century, a number of excellent surgical scientists and surgical achievements have emerged in the western surgical community led by Britain, France, Germany, Italy, and the USA, and there is no forbidden area for surgery—surgeons have been able to enter all body cavities of the human body for surgery. So far, surgery has been separated from manual skills and become an independent science, but the inherent bias and impression of the public about surgery urgently need to be changed.

At the beginning of the twentieth century, William Steward Halsted (1852–1922 A.D.), a famous American surgical scientist directs it to the right path at an important gateway to the development of surgery. He founded the "School of Safe Surgery," emphasizing the safety of surgery, gentle, and careful operation and abandoning the "handsome surgical techniques" previously pursued, and he believed that the fine surgery of 4 or 5 h with gentle operation and careful hemostasis was far less invasive than the aggressive half-hour surgery. In addition, he advocated wearing latex gloves, highly advocated the standardization and systematization of surgical education, and trained a number of excellent surgeons.

Since then, surgeons have gradually gained recognition and their socioeconomic status has increased correspondingly, but there is still confusion about professional functions at that time. During World War I, the US Military Review Board found that more than 50% of ophthalmic examiners did not have professional literacy in ophthalmology. In order to meet the needs of surgical specialty division and professional literacy review standards, the USA has successively established review committees for ophthalmology, orthopedic surgery, colorectal surgery, urology, plastic surgery, surgery, and neurosurgery. The development of American surgery in the twentieth century affected the world. After decades of continuous improvement, the standardization and specialization of surgery were basically completed; in the evaluation system of the public, surgical scientists also officially got rid of the name of manual technicians and became veritable scientists, which can be seen from the list of surgeons who won the Nobel Prize in Physiology or Medicine in the twentieth century (Table 2.1).

1.3.2 Innovation of Surgical Instruments and Imaging Technology

Surgery depends not only on the surgeon's surgical skills, but also on the development of surgical aids. Great advances in science and technology in the twentieth century have led to dramatic changes in medical devices and imaging technology.

The method of burning hemostasis has long been applied in the history of surgical development, but it often has rough means and serious tissue damage. In 1928, the American plant physiologist William T. Bovie (1882–1958 A.D.) invented the high-frequency electrotome, marking the advent of this era of electrosurgery. According to its basic principle, electrosurgery is developed and subdivided into unipolar and bipolar electrosurgery to meet the needs of different types of surgery. Since then, different types of electrosurgical devices such as harmonic scalpel, Ligasure vessel sealing system, argon knife, energy platform, radiofrequency knife, and plasma knife have sprung up, reducing intraoperative bleeding and tissue damage at the technical level.

Table 2.1 Surgeons who won the Nobel Prize in Physiology or Medicine

Prize winner	Nationality	Year of award	Dates of birth and death	Study area
Emil Theodor Kocher	Switzerland	1909	1841–1917	Disorder thyroid
Allvar Gullstrand	Sweden	1911	1862–1930	Ocular refraction
Alexis Carrel	France	1912	1873–1944	Vascular suture and organ transplantation
Robert Bárány	Austria	1914	1876–1936	Vestibular physiology and pathology
Frederick Grant Banting	Canada	1923	1891–1941	Artificial insulin
Anthony Walter Hess	Portugal	1949	1874–1955	Psychosurgery
Werner Forssmann	Germany	1956	1904–1979	Cardiac catheter
Charles Brenton Huggins	Canada	1966	1901–1997	Oncology
Joseph Murray	USA	1990	1919–2012	Human organs and cell transplantation

Before the birth of medical imaging, surgeons could only diagnose diseases based on symptoms and physical examination. Medical imaging equipment has greatly changed the face of clinical diagnosis and laid the foundation for subsequent navigation and interventional procedures. X-ray was used for imaging and disease diagnosis shortly after they were discovered by the German physicist Wilhelm Conrad Röntgen (1845–1923 A.D.) in 1895. In the 1970s, the British electronics engineer Hounsfield, Godfrey Newbold (1919–2004 A.D.) invented CT (computed tomography) and won the 1979 Nobel Prize in Physiology and Medicine. Compared to X-rays, CT takes multiple layers of X-ray images and reconstructs them to obtain images with greater information content, even comparable to surgical dissection. The physical phenomenon of nuclear magnetic resonance was proposed in the 1940s, and magnetic resonance imaging (MRI) technology was applied in the medical field more than 30 years later: in the late 1970s, a 0.15 T magnet up to 1 m long was introduced, and the first human cranial magnetic resonance image was obtained on December 3, 1980. MRI has a high spatial resolution and acquires more anatomical information than CT, gaining competitive development from various countries. The development of ultrasound (US) has benefited from the radar and sonar technology that emerged in the World War II. After simple A-mode ultrasonography and B-mode ultrasonography that can provide cross-sectional dynamics, color Doppler flow imaging is currently used more frequently in clinical practice. Since then, digital subtraction angiography (DSA), single-photon emission computed tomography (SPECT), and positron emission tomography (PET) and other related technologies have been continuously developed, and the system of medical imaging equipment has become increasingly complete.

1.3.3 Development of Minimally Invasive Surgery Concept

Throughout the history of surgery, the surgeon's efforts can be summarized as: trying to complete the procedure or treatment without causing unacceptable injury to the patient. The concept of "minimally invasive" actually always existed. By the twentieth century, the concept of minimally invasive surgery was gradually clarified. Represented by the fact that laparoscopic cholecystectomy was first completed by French physicians in Lyon in 1987, minimally invasive surgery has gradually entered the horizon.

The concept of minimally invasive surgery was not opposed to traditional surgery, and the degree of "minimally invasive" was closely related to the development of science and technology at that time. Minimally invasive surgery is a broader concept than "lumpectomy," "small incisions," "small pathways," "endoscopy," etc. The term "minimally invasive" places more emphasis on causing the least trauma to the body while accomplishing the same goal and is not limited to the modalities or instruments used. Minimally invasive surgery not only meets the patient's pursuit of small incision, but also effectively reduces the patient's surgical injury. Taking malignant tumors as example, laparoscopic exploration avoids huge incisions, greatly reduces the pain of patients, and also strives for valuable time for the subsequent treatment of patients.

Today's surgery is minimally invasive, delicate, and intelligent, as a continuation of laparoscopic technology—robotic surgery is prospering day by day. After the research and development of several generations of robots by several companies, the da Vinci surgical robot developed by American Intuitive Surgery Company was certified by the US FDA in 2000 and has achieved great success in the market. The da Vinci robot greatly improves the speed accuracy of surgery due to its higher magnification, 3D field of view, and flexible and stable robotic hands and joints. As of 2017, 69 machines have been installed in mainland China; the author has used Da Vinci robot to complete hepatobiliary and pancreatic surgery since 2012 (Fig. 2.1), and more than 1800 cases have been completed by 2017. The author realized that

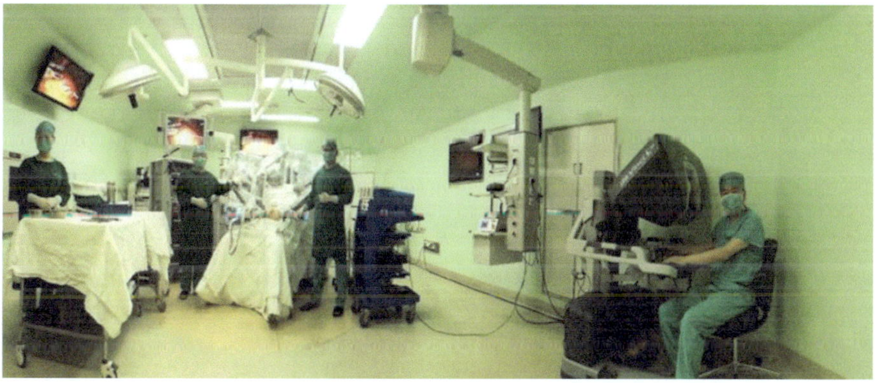

Fig. 2.1 Da Vinci robotic system

there was no significant difference in the incidence rate of postoperative complications compared with laparoscopic surgery.

Surgery has entered the post-minimally invasive surgical era represented by laparoscopic surgery and robotic surgery, but the core of the concept of minimally invasive surgery should not be ignored, not for the sake of "minimally invasive (small incision)," but to truly consider the patient as a whole and make rational decisions based on the evaluation criteria of minimal damage while completing the surgery.

Throughout the history of surgery development, surgery has always been a discipline that closely follows the cutting-edge development of science and technology at that time, rather than unchanged. Surgeons, however, always face different surgical risks around surgery, some of which have been annihilated in the long history, and some of which have not yet been completely solved. The general direction of current surgical development is not simply limited to dealing with problems that have already occurred, not even just early surgery and treatment, but should "cure the disease before it happens," the era of prognosis control surgery is close at hand.

2 Principle of Surgical Risk Management

Surgical diagnosis and treatment is a treatment method centered on a series of invasive operations such as surgery, and its concept should be to save lives, preserve functions, and stop the expansion of injuries, rather than simply the completion of a surgery. Compared with other treatment means, surgical diagnosis and treatment not only faces the threat from the disease, but also is affected by the "side effects" brought about by the surgical operation itself, which often has more direct and serious risks. The development process of surgery can be said to be a history of blood and tears on how to reduce the risk of surgery. More importantly, after the bad results are caused, the surgeons will seek the causes for improvement. However, due to the limitations of the times, surgeons have taken many detours. Up to now, several scientific and technological revolutions have brought us great power for human development, and the crystallization of wisdom contained in them has greatly promoted the diagnosis and treatment ideas and technical progress. Today, surgery should no longer "proceed without a plan," with the mentality of "it is not too late to mend the fold," do a good job of "surgical risk pre-control" to really prevent the occurrence and development of injuries is the core idea of future surgical development.

2.1 Concept and Connotation

In the Yellow Emperor's Classic of Internal Medicine [1], it is said that "the top doctors pay attention to preventive treatment of diseases, but not the existing one." It means that interventions should be made when the disease is not onset or spreading to prevent it before it happens while waiting for the disease to attack and then treating it would be a fallback. Since then, Sun Simiao (541–682 A.D.), a famous doctor of the Tang Dynasty mentioned in his book "Valuable Prescriptions for Emergency" [2] that "the top doctor heals the sickness that is not yet sick; the ordinary doctor heals the sickness that wants to be sick; the low-level doctor heals the sickness that is already sick." By classifying diseases into "not yet sick," "wanting to be sick," and "already sick," it is pointed out that a good doctor can diagnose and treat diseases at an early stage before they occur, so as to prevent them from occurring; an average doctor can control and cure diseases in time when the symptoms of diseases gradually appear; and a low-level doctor can only find out the signs of diseases and remedy them when they are fully developed and become obvious. In fact, the ancient Chinese sages have already put forward the advanced model of medical development—"treating the disease before it happens," which includes two meanings, i.e. to prevent the disease before it happens and to prevent the disease before it changes, called "treating" the disease, but in fact the focus is on "preventing," thus it can be seen that the idea of preventing the disease has already been done. However, since the birth of surgery, surgeons seem to have fallen into some kind of circle of thinking, taking "resection" as the outline and aggressively "transforming" the patient. The inertia of surgeons leads to problems that often arise before they begin to be addressed, with the bloody lessons of history still fresh in our minds. In the concept of medicine, disease refers to disease and illness, and specifically in surgery, the "disease" that needs to be "treated" or "prevented" is actually the risk associated with surgical operations. Today's surgeons, especially those in primary care, still generally lack awareness of surgical risk prevention and are still deficient in the skilled use of scientific methods and technical tools to deal with surgical risks. The author advocates to apply risk pre-control theory, grasp the use of scientific risk pre-control system, and systematically respond to and handle surgical risks.

Surgical risk pre-control theory refers to the risk identification and risk assessment of potential surgical risks that have not occurred and further measures are taken for risk prevention, as well as timely risk control of surgical risks that have occurred, in order to avoid the occurrence of risks or reduce the risk of injury. The key core of solving surgical risks and doing a good job in risk pre-control lies in paying attention to cultivating the awareness of surgical risk pre-control, scientifically using the existing technical means, summarizing the lessons learned from theory and practice, and forming a complete surgical risk pre-control system (Fig. 2.2).

2.2 Surgical Risk Pre-control System

The main contents of surgical risk pre-control system include two parts.

The first is risk identification, assessment, and prevention. Before a risk occurs, the surgeon should anticipate potential risks, understand which risks are likely to occur, conduct a systematic assessment of the likely risks, determine the severity of the consequences of the risk, and finally take steps to eliminate the risk or reduce the likelihood of the risk occurring.

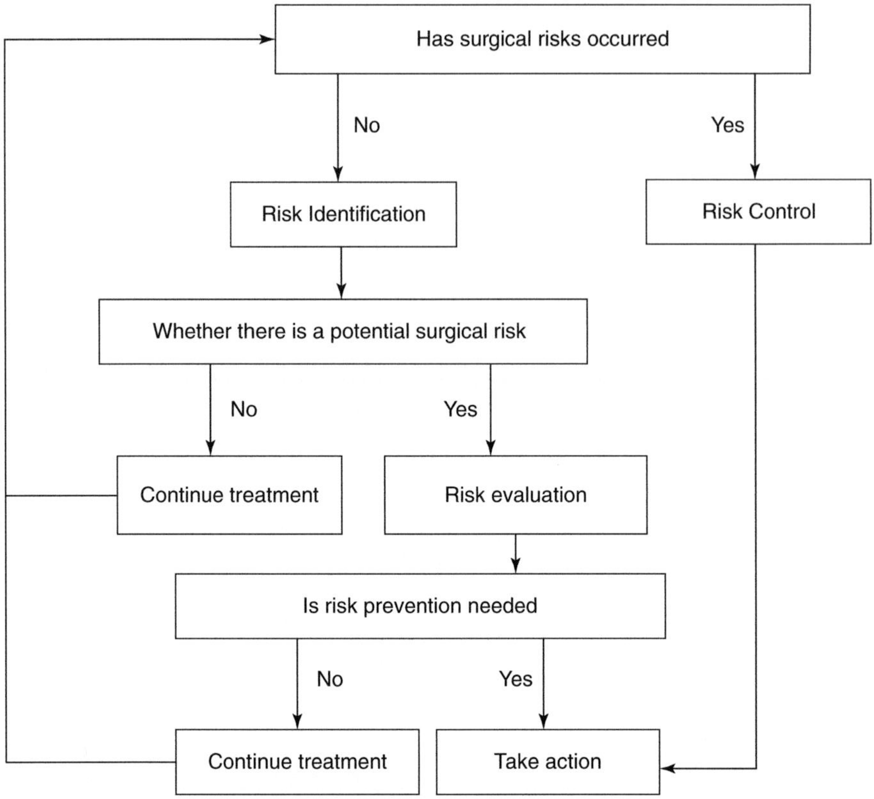

Fig. 2.2 Flow chart of surgical risk pre-control

The second is risk control. In case of any risk, it is necessary to immediately make intervention, cut off the development chain of risk, and timely handle the adverse consequences already caused, so as to minimize the damage. After the completion of risk handling, the handling scheme shall be summarized and continuously improved, and the scheme shall be adopted to transform high risks into low risks, so as to truly prevent problems before they occur.

2.2.1 Risk Identification, Evaluation, and Prevention

Risk Identification

Risk identification is the first step in the overall risk prevention process and refers to the process by which surgeons make a pre-judgment about potential risks. On the one hand, this can be roughly judged through the accumulated experience of doctors. On the other hand, it is more important to analyze, summarize, and evaluate the specific conditions by using the principle of evidence-based medicine and combining with the existing risk evaluation system, so as to predict whether the surgical risks may occur and summarize the reasons and rules for the occurrence of risks. The elements of risk identification include risk events, risk factors and adverse consequences, which focus on grasping the reasons and conditions for the occurrence of risks and the nature of risks themselves.

The process of risk identification is the most difficult step in the risk pre-control process, which requires not only an ultra-clear understanding of the principles of surgical risk occurrence and development, but also a meticulous observation and comprehensive understanding of specific cases, and finally a scientific risk analysis and prediction method.

Risk Evaluation

Risk evaluation refers to that on the basis of risk identification, based on widely recognized evidence-based medical evidence, using the existing auxiliary examination means and risk evaluation scale, using the statistical method to systematically and objectively assess the possible surgical risks, evaluate their severity, and provide the basis for the next step of risk prevention.

The process of risk evaluation is very complex, and quantitative analysis is usually required. Under the special background that medicine is difficult to accurately quantify, there are many limitations in the process of risk evaluation. The surgeon should take a sound risk assessment approach, combining validity, reliability, and ease of use. Risk evaluation can help surgeons correctly evaluate the advantages and disadvantages of surgical treatment. The overall benefit of the treatment taken for the patients is the greatest, rather than waste food due to choking.

Risk identification and risk evaluation are necessary contents for risk prevention, while prediction is “quantitative” and evaluation is “quantity.” Both complement each other and are interrelated: only when the existence of risk is predicted, the risk can be further evaluated consciously and purposefully. Only through risk identification and assessment, the various factors leading to the occurrence of surgical risks can be identified, serving the proposed risk prevention options and assisting clinical decision-making.

Risk Prevention

Risk prevention refers to the specific measures taken to avoid, eliminate, and reduce the losses caused by surgical risks before they occur, with the focus on reducing risk factors to reduce the probability of loss occurrence. There are no restrictions on the specific forms or measures of risk prevention, including changing the surgical approach, improving surgical skills, adjusting medication regimens, and even reasonable doctor–patient communication, which can be the direction of surgeons' efforts as long as it helps to reduce the occurrence of risks.

The long-term goal of risk prevention is to form a complete risk early warning system. In addition to reasonable medical norms to maximize the subjective initiative of surgeons, the use of emerging and newly developed high-tech means can achieve real-time monitoring of the patient's condition and the treatment behavior of surgical staff and strangle surgical risks in the embryonic stage.

2.2.2 Risk Control

When surgical risks have occurred, it means that the means of risk prevention have been ineffective. At this time, it is necessary to immediately change ideas and decisively adopt patterned intervention means to limit injury at an early stage and interrupt the risk development chain; strictly consider other treatment measures that may increase injury, so as to avoid further expansion of injury.

The concept of damage control has been proposed in the 1970s, but it is mainly applicable to patients who receive severe trauma. The purpose is mainly not to further aggravate the injury, resulting in the situation that the gains and losses of "the operation are completed and the people are gone." The author believes that in the face of general surgical risks, the concept of early detection and decisive treatment is more applicable, while in the face of severe trauma, it is more practical to avoid risk expansion and control the risk in a small range.

At the same time, intervention optimization should be achieved, that is, treatment means should be continuously improved in the process of risk pre-control to control the severity of adverse consequences within the minimum range. After a treatment event, all the processes should be summarized and discussed, the treatment process should be repeatedly optimized, and the risk should be faced methodically again to achieve the best effect. Intervention optimization measures are based on two points, experience, that is, continuously summarizing experience after the occurrence of risk, and then summarizing into theory; literature, mainly relying on learning the literature with higher level of evidence-based medicine evidence, does not rely on the surgical risks seen by the surgeon. Combining the two organically can achieve better risk control.

Surgical risk pre-control theory is a thought system to correctly cope with surgical risks, and its main contents include risk identification, risk evaluation, risk prevention, damage control, and intervention optimization. It focuses on "prognosis" and takes into account "control." The core purpose is to strangle the risk when it does not occur. The following chapters will detail the various aspects of risk pre-control theory with a view to providing the surgical professional reader with a methodology for the rational management of surgical risks.

3 Surgical Risk Identification

Surgical risks exist objectively in the whole process of surgical diagnosis and treatment, with the characteristics of difficult to detect in advance and serious consequences once they occur. Simply put, to prevent risks, it is necessary to first clarify whether there is a risk, and this is risk identification. Whether the risk identification is comprehensive and correct is the key to decide whether surgical risks can be successfully prevented. Successful risk identification involves answering the following questions: What are the surgical risks to be considered? Which individuals will be affected by what? What are the main factors that cause these risks? Risk identification is the first and most important and difficult step of risk pre-control.

3.1 What Is the Surgical Risk Identification?

Case 1: A 70-year-old patient visited the general surgery clinic of a grade A class 3 hospital and complained of abdominal pain and distension with belching for 1 year. Abdominal contrast-enhanced CT showed antral mass without distant metastasis, considering the possibility of malignancy. Past medical history: The patient had myocardial infarction attack for 1 year and received cardiac stent implantation. The patient recovered well after operation and continued to take Warfarin till now; the patient had chronic obstructive pulmonary disease for 10 years, and the condition was stable after drug treatment. He came to the clinic for surgical treatment. After asking medical history, browsing information about the condition and conducting physical examination, the doctor gave the following recommendations: (1) After stopping anticoagulant drugs for 1 week, check the four coagulation items, and after the indicators are not significantly abnormal, consult our department for surgical treatment; (2) Joint consultation of cardiology, respiratory medicine, and anesthesiology to improve the preoperative evaluation.

The above is a very common treatment process in the general surgery clinic of the hospital, but the surgeon made a very reasonable judgment according to the patient's condition and in combination with his own experience: since the patient took anticoagulant drugs, which is a contraindication for surgery, it is necessary to discontinue the drug for 1 week and check whether the coagulation function is abnormal before surgical treatment; in addition, due to the patient's history of heart disease and lung disease, it is necessary to cooperate with the relevant departments for preoperative evaluation to determine whether the patient can tolerate the surgery. In this case, the surgeon identified that the patient had risks of intraoperative bleeding and cardiopulmonary accident and used reasonable strategies to deal with it. From the above case, it can be seen that risk identification is not out of reach, but is always applied in surgical clinical practice and has a significant impact on the decision of clinical treatment plan.

The identification of surgical risks means that, before the risks cause adverse consequences, the surgeon comprehensively, continuously, and objectively judges and analyzes to determine whether the patient may have surgical risks, the types and sources of potential surgical risks, recognizes various surgical risks, and summarizes and regularly analyzes the dynamic process of causes of surgical risks (Fig. 2.3). The relevant elements of surgical risk identification mainly include various surgical risk events, risk factors, and adverse consequences. Risk factors are defined as the conditions or events that may increase the frequency or severity of surgical risks.

3.2 How Is Surgical Risk Identification Performed?

The purpose of surgical risk identification is to systematically analyze and provide a basic description of the causes of risk, drivers of risk, risk events, and possible adverse consequences. Its main contents include:

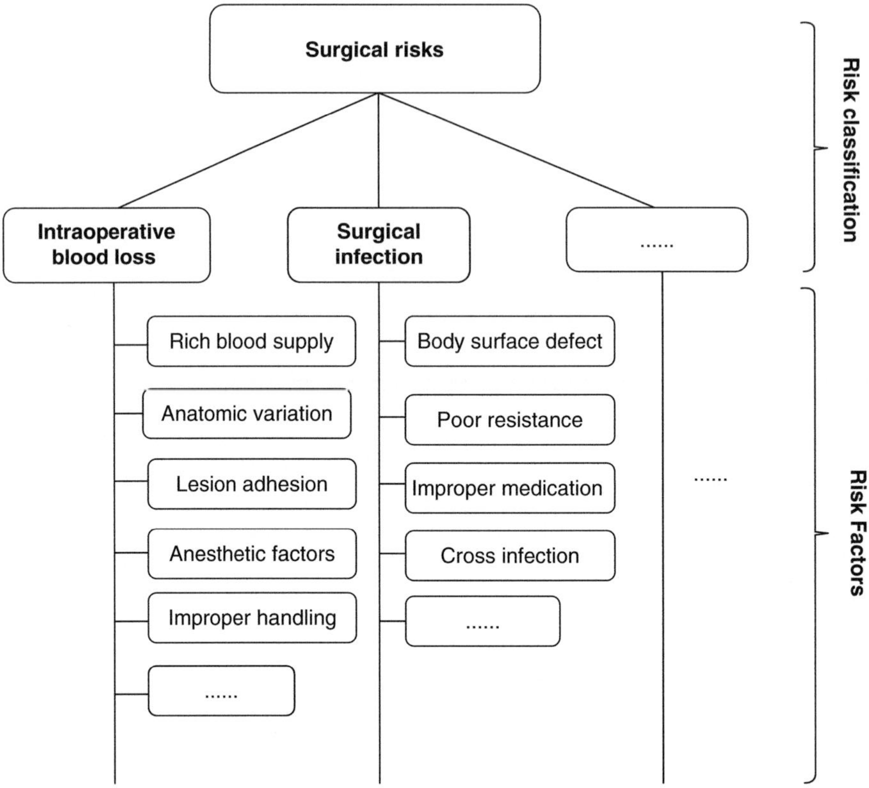

Fig. 2.3 Logic tree diagram of surgical risk identification

1. To understand surgical risk rationale. Medicine is a discipline that attaches equal importance to theory and practice. Surgeons need to correctly understand surgical risks based on their previous medical knowledge, theory, and practical experience. In Case 1, the surgeon correctly judged that this patient was temporarily not suitable for surgery due to "learned" and "seen" similar conditions.
2. To master the risk occurrence environment. After having the theoretical and empirical basis, it is also necessary to have a thorough understanding of the environment in which surgical risks occur, such as the patient's condition and the doctor–patient communication environment, and to combine theoretical experience with the actual situation of the individual patient. Understanding the principles of surgical risk occurrence and development and mastering the occurrence environment of surgical risks are the basis for surgical risk identification, and the above two works can also be called building a risk prevention environment.
3. To analyze surgical risk factors. The contents mainly include the analysis of various causes and conditions that may cause surgical risks and mastering the risk factors that cause adverse consequences. The study of risk factors has always been a hot issue for surgeons, but the analysis of risk factors in most studies is

cluttered and often omission occurs. Taking surgery-related risks as the research object, according to the method of surgical risk identification, surgical risk factors can be macroscopically divided into objective factors (not affected by external conditions and physician behaviors) and subjective factors (affected by other conditions), which can be specifically divided into disease factors, physiological factors, systemic factors, and operating factors (see below for specific definition). By analyzing the risk factors according to the above classification method, it can help readers to comprehensively and rationally analyze the risk factors.

Case 2: A 70-year-old male patient. The patient was admitted due to "painless progressive icteric skin and sclera for 2 weeks." Physical examination: T: 36.2 °C, P: 71 bpm, BP: 160/105 mmHg. The skin and sclera were yellowish, and an enlarged liver and gallbladder were palpable in the right upper quadrant. Murphy's sign (−). Laboratory tests showed that total bilirubin 271 μmol/L, direct bilirubin 185 μmol/L, γ-GT 1124 U/L, alanine aminotransferase 311 U/L, aspartate aminotransferase 159 U/L, CA19–91211 U/mL, and CEA 6.94 μg/L. Pancreatic MRI + enhancement: intrahepatic and extrahepatic bile duct dilatation, pancreatic head mass, considering malignant tumor. Preoperative examination was planned to be completed and elective pancreaticoduodenectomy was performed.

In the case shown in Case 2, it is necessary to analyze the risk factors that may cause intraoperative bleeding. Is it due to the difficulty in performing the complex local anatomy of the pancreatic head? Is the patient complicated with jaundice and poor coagulation function? Or the patient's history of hypertension, intraoperative blood pressure may be poorly controlled? This requires the surgeon to identify possible surgical risk factors in combination with existing professional knowledge, experience, and the actual condition of the patient and also paves the way for further risk evaluation and prevention.

In clinical practice, surgeons face a variety of surgical risks, and the risk factors causing adverse outcomes include both objective factors such as factors of the disease itself and subjective factors of both doctors and patients (Chap. 1, Sect. 2). The following features are especially considered in the process of risk identification.

The first is integrity. The human body is a whole, and "pull one hair and the whole body is affected." Surgeons should not be limited to their own "acre of land," but should take a holistic view of the condition and identify surgical risks in a comprehensive manner. As in Case 1, the surgeon comprehensively considers the patient's heart and lung diseases, rather than just focusing on gastric tumors and rushing to perform surgery.

The second is continuity. The patient's condition is in a dynamic process. As the disease progresses and the treatment intervenes, the quality and quantity of previous potential surgical risks have been changing, and new surgical risks may also occur. It is difficult for surgeons to identify the full range of surgical risks faced by their patients without continuous observation and analysis of the patients.

The third is procedure. Risk identification, as a scientific derivation and analysis behavior, needs to be run by the organization, constrained by the system, and performed according to established procedures and processes. It is inevitable that a surgeon will have omissions in comprehensive and objective analysis, so it is necessary for the diagnosis and treatment group or even multidisciplinary discussion to strictly implement the three-level ward round system and preoperative discussion system in order to improve the rationality and accuracy of identification.

3.3 Analysis of Risk Factors for Common Surgical Risks

3.3.1 Intraoperative Bleeding

Intraoperative bleeding refers to intraoperative arteriovenous rupture caused by various reasons, which has no obvious adverse consequences after effective control, but if the amount of bleeding is too much, it can further cause hemorrhagic shock or even death. Any surgeon will face the risk of intraoperative bleeding, and the specific risk factors causing intraoperative bleeding vary greatly according to the surgical procedure.

The main risk factors of bleeding during cesarean section include uterine atony, incision factors, placental factors, and coagulation dysfunction, with different specific causes. The risk factors of bleeding during cesarean section are summarized and the specific causes are analyzed (Table 2.2).

The risk identification method is used to analyze it. Except that "too small and too low uterine incision" is a subjective factor, the rest are objective factors.

1. Disease factors.

   They refer to the risk factors caused by local pathological changes of disease itself or lesions. For bleeding during cesarean section, risk factors due to the disease itself include: prolonged labor, polyhydramnios, anemia, uterine apoplexy, intrauterine infection, uterine fibroids, placenta previa, placenta accreta, placental adhesion, placental abruption, retained placenta, amniotic fluid embolism, severe placental abruption. Although pregnancy is a normal physiological process in the above case, it can be secondary to a variety of pathological processes causing intraoperative bleeding. Among other surgical diseases, local

Table 2.2 Risk factors for bleeding during cesarean section

Risk factors	Specific causes
Uterine contractions weak	Prolonged labor; polyhydramnios, multiple pregnancy, macrosomia; pregnancy-induced hypertension, anemia, placental abruption, uterine apoplexy, intrauterine infection, uterine fibroids
Incision factors	Too small and too low uterine incision, too large fetal head, too low fetal head embedded in the pelvic cavity; local compression tissue edema due to prolonged labor
Placental factors	Placenta previa, placenta accreta, placental adhesion, placental abruption, retained placenta (history of miscarriage, induced labor, pelvic inflammatory disease can increase risk)
Coagulation dysfunction	Severe pregnancy-induced hypertension, HELLP syndrome, amniotic fluid embolism, severe placental abruption, liver function damage, hematological diseases

abnormalities, local adhesions, and local anatomical abnormalities are also disease risk factors for intraoperative bleeding.

2. Physiological factors.

   They refer to the risk factors not caused by pathological process, but generated by its own physiological conditions. Physiological factors for bleeding during cesarean section include: multiple pregnancies, too large fetal head, and too low fetal head embedded in the pelvic cavity. The physiological factors of intraoperative bleeding risk are objective factors for the occurrence of risk and usually include local anatomical variation, location of the lesion, and abundant blood supply to the focal organ. Since some physiological factors already exist before the operation is performed, the surgeon can analyze them in detail before the operation and make a good understanding.

3. Systemic factors.

   They refer to the risk factors of other organs, systems, or systemic risk factors caused by diseases or other reasons. The physiological factors of bleeding during cesarean section include: pregnancy-induced hypertension, anemia, HELLP syndrome, liver function damage, and hematological diseases. Specifically, systemic factors include both secondary changes caused by the disease itself and the patient's comorbidities.

4. Iatrogenic factors.

   They refer to the risk factors caused by the surgeon's own technical or operational reasons and diagnosis and treatment conditions. The operative factor for intraoperative bleeding during cesarean delivery is a too small and low uterine incision. Risk factors such as improper preoperative planning and intraoperative violent operation among operating factors should be avoided as much as possible. It should be noted that several other factors are often able to increase the possibility of surgical risk caused by iatrogenic factors, which the author calls "forced errors." As you can imagine, the best surgeons still cannot completely avoid intraoperative bleeding due to inherent factors such as anatomical variants and intraoperative adhesions, so surgical risks due to medical factors, although they can be reduced, cannot be completely avoided. However, careful preoperative understanding of the patient's condition, good surgical planning, and gentle intraoperative handling should still be the direction of the surgeon's relentless pursuit of technical excellence.

Liver surgery also faces a serious threat of intraoperative bleeding. As an important parenchymal organ of the human body, the liver is supplied by the hepatic artery and portal venous system. The main hepatic vein and short hepatic vein collect hepatic blood flow and drain into the veins. At the same time, there are also a large number of communicating branches between the liver and the surrounding organ tissues. Intraoperative bleeding in liver surgery has always been one of the difficult problems for surgeons. Chen XP summarized 4368 cases of hepatectomy, of which 286 cases had intraoperative bleeding, mainly due to macrovascular injury, liver cirrhosis-portal hypertension, poor liver function, and extensive adhesion of the tumor to the surrounding organs. The specific bleeding causes are shown in Table 2.3.

Table 2.3 Causes of major bleeding during hepatectomy ($n = 286$)

Causes of bleeding	Number of cases	%
Injury of main hepatic vein	23	8.0
Vena cava injury	2	0.7
Injury of short hepatic vein	19	6.7
Variceal rupture in the first porta hepatis	28	9.8
Hepatic section bleeding	29	10.1
Diaphragmatic wound bleeding	36	12.6
Tumor rupture	23	8.0
Extensive adhesion around tumor	126	44.1
Total	286	100

According to the method of surgical risk identification, we can also classify the risk factors of intraoperative bleeding in hepatectomy: tumor rupture and extensive adhesion around the tumor are disease factors; main hepatic vein injury, vena cava injury, and short hepatic vein injury are operation factors; while variceal rupture in the first porta hepatis, hepatic section bleeding, and diaphragmatic wound bleeding may be related to the local pathological state caused by disease factors, systemic factors such as coagulation abnormalities and operation factors of surgeons.

Intraoperative bleeding is a common problem during surgery, and there are many causes of intraoperative bleeding, which may sometimes be influenced by a combination of risk factors. Overall, intraoperative bleeding may not be completely avoided, but the risk factors are relatively clear. Mastering the principle of risk occurrence and scientific risk identification method can comprehensively and correctly understand the risk factors and lay a foundation for effectively reducing the probability of intraoperative bleeding.

3.3.2 Surgical Infection

Surgical infections usually refer to infectious diseases requiring surgical treatment and surgery-related infections. When studying surgical risks, we mainly study surgical site infection (SSI) and analyze its risk factors using risk identification methods.

In 1999, the Centers for Disease Control and Prevention first defined SSI and issued guidelines for SSI prevention, which were clinically recognized. SSIs are the most common surgical infections and are defined as those that occur at the surgical site and can be divided into three categories by definition: (1) superficial SSIs, which are infections of the skin and subcutaneous tissues of the incision; (2) deep SSIs, which progress to the deep layers of the incision, including the muscles and fascia; and (3) organ/space SSIs, which include abdominal abscesses, empyema, and joint space infections. Based on the results of a large number of clinical cases, a number of studies have analyzed the risk factors for SSI, and the author summarizes them in combination with his own experience as follows (Table 2.4).

Table 2.4 Risk factors for surgical site infection

Risk factors	Specific reason
Objective factors	
Patient's own factors	Age, obesity, preoperative malnutrition, underlying diseases (diabetes, COPD, etc.), malignancy, liver cirrhosis, AIDS, skin diseases
Non-patient factors	Surgical site, hospital stay, presence/absence of implant, incision type/grade
Subjective factors	Use of prophylactic antibiotics
	Surgeon specific infection rate Preoperative skin preparation Improper skin disinfection Length of operation Waiting time for surgery Surgical tips and suturing techniques Surgical method Operating room environment Intraoperative factors: Hypothermia, etc.

We can still categorize risk factors according to standard risk identification methods:

1. Disease factors

   These include surgical site, hospital stay, incision type/grade.
2. Physiological factors

   It mainly refers to patient's age.
3. Systemic factors

   These include obesity, preoperative malnutrition, diabetes, COPD, malignant tumors, cirrhosis, AIDS, skin diseases, and the presence or absence of implants.
4. Iatrogenic factors

   The use of prophylactic antibiotics, surgeon specific infection rate, preoperative skin preparation, improper skin disinfection, operation time, waiting time for operation, hospital stay, surgical skills and suture techniques, surgical methods, operating room environment, and intraoperative hypothermia are iatrogenic factors.

3.3.3 Digestive Tract Fistula

Digestive tract fistula included internal fistula and external fistula, according to the location of injury can be divided into gastric fistula, intestinal fistula, pancreatic fistula, biliary fistula, and so on. Digestive tract fistula is one of the common complications of abdominal surgery, which not only affects the surgical effect; especially for patients with malignant tumors, it is often associated with malnutrition, abdominal infection and internal environment disorders caused by digestive tract fistula can even endanger the patient's life. In order to reduce the incidence of digestive tract fistula, abdominal surgeons have conducted a large number of related studies on risk factors, which are summarized by the author in combination with his own clinical experience in the following table (Table 2.5).

Table 2.5 Risk factors of postoperative gastrointestinal fistula

Type	Risk factors
Gastrointestinal/ anastomotic fistula	Age, obesity, anemia, combined intestinal obstruction, combined diabetes, preoperative albumin level, preoperative hemoglobin level, neoadjuvant chemotherapy, surgical methods/resection range, digestive tract reconstruction methods, anastomosis technique, abdominal drainage tube placement
Pancreatic fistula	Age, obesity, anemia, combined diabetes, preoperative albumin level, preoperative hemoglobin level, preoperative total bilirubin, neoadjuvant chemoradiotherapy, history of abdominal surgery, operation time, intraoperative blood loss, main pancreatic duct diameter, pancreatic texture, pancreaticojejunostomy, pancreatic duct support tube drainage, postoperative application of somatostatin analogues
Biliary fistula	Age, obesity, anemia, combined diabetes, preoperative albumin level, preoperative hemoglobin level, preoperative total bilirubin, neoadjuvant chemoradiotherapy, history of abdominal surgery, operation time, intraoperative blood loss, bile duct diameter, liver section area, method and technique of choledochojejunostomy

There are many risk factors of digestive tract fistula, some of which have obtained international consensus. It is easy to classify risk into objective and subjective risk factors according to the method of risk identification, which can be further summarized as follows:

1. Disease factors

   These include the diameter of the main pancreatic duct, the texture of the pancreas, and the diameter of the bile duct.
2. Physiological factors

   They mainly refer to the patient's age and fat and thin.
3. Systemic factors

   These include obesity, anemia, combined intestinal obstruction, combined diabetes, history of abdominal surgery, preoperative albumin level, preoperative hemoglobin level, and neoadjuvant chemotherapy.
4. Iatrogenic factors

   Surgical methods, resection range, operation time, intraoperative blood loss, liver section area, digestive tract reconstruction methods, anastomosis techniques, pancreaticojejunostomy methods, pancreatic duct support tube drainage methods, abdominal drainage tube placement, postoperative application of somatostatin analogues, choledochojejunostomy methods, and techniques are iatrogenic factors.

Risk identification is the first step in the overall surgical risk pre-control process, which refers to the process of judging, classifying, clarifying, and overall analyzing the potential surgical risks faced by risk subjects (especially patients). On the one hand, the identification of risks is judged through the learned knowledge and accumulated experience; on the other hand, it is also necessary to rely on objective risk analysis, induction, and arrangement to finally complete the identification of the possible adverse consequences of various surgical risks as well as the law of risk occurrence. Risk identification is a continuous and systematic effort. Since a large number of new conditions, new complications, and accidents occur during the whole process from treatment, hospitalization to surgery, and discharge, these conditions either increase new risks or change the degree or nature of original risks. This requires the surgeon to continuously identify, continuously detect changes in the already predicted risks, and new surgical risks that may arise in the future.

4 Surgical Risk Assessment

Before surgery, patients and their family members often ask, "Is the surgery risky?" This really brothers the surgeons. We can articulate the full range of risks that can occur; given the real-world medical climate, surgeons tend to describe each consequence as very serious and often have difficulty giving a probability of occurrence of surgical risk. Patients are often "frightened" and "unable to sleep well over night" after receiving such information, and some patients even give up the surgery. So what is the actual probability that a surgical risk will occur? How serious are the consequences? Can surgical risks to the patient be graded or quantified? The above questions can be answered upon completion of the surgical risk evaluation.

4.1 Overview of Surgical Risk Evaluation

Surgical risk evaluation refers to the evaluation and estimation of the probability and severity of surgical risks based on the existing practice-tested theory and various evaluation scales or consensus guidelines, using the method of statistical analysis, on the basis of risk identification, to provide the basis for risk prevention.

Risk evaluation is a very difficult and complicated work, because it must be combined with the probability of risk and the severity of the consequences (i.e. losses) of two factors, and then the same scale to measure, in order to determine the magnitude of losses caused by risks. In surgical practice, although the severity of consequences can be determined by the same scale, it is difficult to accurately quantify. Similar to that the condition of inpatients can only be generally divided into critical, severe, and general. Various risk evaluation tables can only score and grade the risks. The fine quantitative analysis of adverse consequences is still difficult to achieve. Conversely, due to the particularity of medicine, there are many variables that affect the consequences, and there is a quantitative analysis prediction method for the probability of risk occurrence only when it targets some surgical risks, even so it cannot be very accurate. Overall, despite many limitations, surgical risk evaluation is still an indispensable step in the surgical risk pre-control system, which establishes the risk pre-control system on the framework of scientific and quantitative analysis and provides a more reliable theoretical basis for the final completion of risk pre-control.

As shown in Table 2.6, the anesthesia grading (ASA), surgical incision cleanliness, estimated surgery duration, and surgical category are clear and scored from low to high. However, the surgical risk evaluation is relatively simple on the mathematical statistics of whether there should be a difference of 1 point between adjacent grades and whether the total NNIS score should be simply added. As mentioned

Table 2.6 Surgical risk assessment table

Anesthesia grading (ASA grading)	P1	A normal patient; no systemic disease other than localized disease	0□
	P2	A patient with minor clinical symptoms; mild or severe systemic disease	0□
	P3	A patient with a severe systemic disease that limits activity but is not incapacitating	1□
	P4	A patient with an incapacitating severe systemic disease that is a constant threat to life	1□
	P5	A moribund patient who is not expected to survive	1□
	P6	A patient with brain death	1□
Signature of anesthesiologist	Date:		
Surgical incision cleanliness	Class I surgical incision (clean surgery)	• No contamination of surgical field; no inflammation around the surgical incision • Patients do not have airway, esophageal, and/or urethral catheterization • Patients have no disturbance of consciousness	0□
	Class II surgical incision (relatively clean surgery)	• Surgery of upper and lower respiratory tract, upper and lower gastrointestinal tract, genitourinary tract, or above organs • Patients are intubated with airway, esophagus, and/or urethra • Patients are in stable conditions • Patients undergo gallbladder, vaginal, appendiceal, ear and nose surgery	0□
	Class III surgical incision (clean-contaminated surgery)	• Open, fresh, and dirty wounds • Infected incision after previous surgery • Incision requiring disinfection during surgery	1□
	Class IV surgical incision (contaminated surgery)	• Severe trauma, inflammation, and tissue necrosis in the surgical incision, or visceral drainage tube	1□
Estimated surgery duration	T1: Surgery is estimated to be completed within 3 h		0□
	T2: Surgery is estimated to be completed in more than 3 h		1□

Table 2.6 (continued)

Surgery category	Superficial tissue surgery	□
	Deep tissue surgery	□
	Organ surgery	□
	Lacunar operation	□
Preoperative NNIS grading	ASA grading of anesthesia + surgical incision cleanliness + surgery duration = 0-□ 1-□ 2-□ 3-□	
Signature of surgeon	Date:	
Is it an emergency surgery	Emergency surgery	□
Actual surgery duration	Surgery completed within 3 h	0□
	Surgery completed over 3 h	1□
Postoperative NNIS grading	ASA grading of anesthesia + surgical incision cleanliness + surgery duration = 0-□ 1-□ 2-□ 3-□	
Signature of circulating nurse	Date:	
Wound healing	Grade A healing □ superficial incision infection □ deep incision infection □ others	
Signature of treating physician	Date:	

earlier, medicine has certain particularities in science, and we cannot calculate the effects of all factors on the results very accurately. However, the relative positions of the different scores do not change, and this "fuzzy" treatment has the advantage of facilitating practical application.

In summary, the author believes that the overall principle of surgical risk evaluation should be to combine comprehensive and scientific findings to summarize risk factors and simple and easy risk grading methods to maximize the subjective initiative of surgeons and to accurately evaluate the risk evaluation level as much as possible under the framework of the current routine preoperative discussion system and multidisciplinary consultation system with the current scope of knowledge.

4.2 Auxiliary Instruments for Surgical Risk Evaluation

Risk assessment is not rootless, and it is possible to make it comprehensive and accurate based on a thorough understanding of the patient's existing signs and symptoms, combined with ancillary examination tests.

4.2.1 General Condition of Patients

The general conditions of patients, including medical history, symptoms, signs, and daily activity status, are directly reflected by the patient's condition and are an important basis for surgical risk evaluation. This information can often be used to quickly understand the patient's condition, and a variety of assessment scales and evaluation methods also include it as an important scoring item. Due to many limitations of current medical level, many auxiliary examinations still cannot accurately evaluate the patient's condition; the collection of relevant information on the patient's medical history, symptoms, signs, and daily activity status is relatively simple and feasible, and the risk evaluation method based on this is also convenient for clinicians to use. Medical history, symptoms, and signs play an absolutely important role in the evaluation of surgical risks.

In Case 1, the assessment of metabolic equivalent is finally determined according to whether the patient can tolerate the corresponding physical activity. Although we can also determine the metabolic equivalent by the results of treadmill exercise test and bicycle exercise test, for the patients with higher metabolic equivalent, the exercise test can be completely not performed. According to the patient's physical activity (self-care activity is the most commonly used), it can be determined that the cardiovascular risk before surgery is lower; for the patients with lower metabolic equivalent, detailed cardiovascular-related examination can be performed, which can effectively save medical resources.

Case 1: In the preoperative cardiovascular risk evaluation of non-cardiac surgery, the most important thing is not electrocardiogram, echocardiography, coronary CT, but metabolic equivalent (MET). As an indicator of relative exercise intensity, metabolic equivalents are basically based on the patient's medical history as a reference, so as to objectively assess the possibility of cardiovascular risk before surgery. Metabolic equivalents are relative measures of the level of energy metabolism during various activities expressed on the basis of energy expenditure in quiet, sitting position. 1 MET is equivalent to 1 kcal per hour per kilogram of body weight (1MET = 1 kcal/kg/h) or 1 MET is equivalent to 3.5 mL of oxygen per minute per kilogram of body weight (1MET = VO2 3.5 mL/kg/min) at absolute rest. In brief, metabolic equivalent refers to the patient's activity tolerance. After screening for cardiovascular instability as described above, by taking a history (ask the following 3 questions): (1) Can you take care of yourself? (2) Do you have chest tightness or shortness of breath when going up 2 stairs? (3) What activities or exercises are usually performed?, this allows a more systematic assessment of the patient's metabolic equivalents. It is classified into 10 levels, with 1 MET representing activities such as dressing and eating, 4 METs representing the ability to climb 2 stairs, and 10 METs representing the ability to play ball, swim, and climb mountains. The following table lists the metabolic equivalents corresponding to some common physical activities (Table 2.7).

It is pointed out in the guidelines of Europe and the USA that even patients with high cardiovascular risk can be operated without other examinations as long as they can easily climb two stairs or more and the metabolic equivalent is greater than 10; for patients with metabolic equivalent greater than 4, other exercise tests and cardiac imaging examinations may still be considered.

4.2.2 Accessory Examination

Auxiliary examinations mainly include laboratory examination, radiology examination, ECG room related examination, CT examination, magnetic resonance examination, nuclear medicine examination, interventional related examination, and

Table 2.7 The metabolic equivalents corresponding to the common physical activities

METs	Self-care activities	Household activities	Recreational activities	Occupational activities
1–2	Bed rest, meals in sitting and standing position, talking, changing clothes and washing face, walking at 1.7 km/h, flying and driving wheelchair in sitting position	Sewing by hand, sweeping, knitting, wiping furniture	TV, radio, chess, painting in sitting position	Transactional work, watch repair, typing, computer operation
2–3	Slower level walking (3.2 km/h), cycling (8 km/h), bedside toilet, riding in standing position	Peel, knead dough, wash small clothes, sweep bed, wipe glass, clean courtyard, machine sewing, laundry tableware	Driving, boating (4 km/h), riding horse slow, playing piano (stringed instrument)	Repair (electrical appliances, shoes), tailor, doorman, nanny, printer, salesman, hotel attendant
3–4	Ordinary level walking (4 km/h), cycling (10 km/h), showering	Make beds, mop the floor, dry clothes by hand, hang clothes, cook	Radio, fishing, playing organ	Taxi driver, tile worker, locksmith, welder, tractor, farmland, machine assembly
4–5	Walking slightly faster on flat ground (5 km/h), cycling (13 km/h), downstairs, bathing	Shopping (light stuff), weed control	Dancing, gardening, playing table tennis, swimming (18.3 m/min)	Light farm work, pasting wallpaper, construction workers (outdoor), carpenters (light work), painters
5–6	Walking fast on flat ground (5.5 km/h), cycling (17.5 km/h)	Ripping, parenting	Riding horse fast, skating (14.5 km/h)	Farm work, carpenter, roadkeeper, coal miner
6–7	Jogging (4–5 km/h), cycling (17.5 km/h)	Chopping wood, sweeping snow	Tennis (singles), light ski	Road repair engineering, cement worker, logging
7–8	Cycling (19 km/h)	Digging trenches with shovels and carrying (<36 kg of heavy objects)	Hiking, galloping on horseback, swimming, skiing, playing basketball	Grazing, planer
8	10 consecutive flights of stairs, jogging (8.9 km/h)	–	Various sports games	Furnaceman (shovel coal >16 kg/min)

pathological examination. Compared with the patient's history, symptoms, signs, and daily activity status as well as the evaluation and judgment made by clinicians based on the above information, the auxiliary examination is more accurate and objective. By using the measurement method of uniform standard, the subjectivity of evaluation can be substantially removed by using the results of auxiliary examination. In terms of practical application, such results are often more recognized (5.2). In surgical risk evaluation, laboratory tests and electrocardiography-related test results are more widely used, and imaging tests are more commonly used in disease diagnosis and surgical planning.

Case 2: Modified Child–Pugh classification: In 1954, Child first proposed the concept of liver function classification, including five factors: serum bilirubin, plasma albumin, ascites, general status, and nutrition, which could quantitatively assess the liver reserve function of patients with cirrhosis; in 1964, the newly proposed Child–Turcotte classification replaced the general status with hepatic encephalopathy, which was relatively simple and practical, forming a classical Child classification; however, due to the subjective evaluation of nutritional status factors, Pugh proposed Child–Turcotte–Pugh classification on the basis of the original classification shortly thereafter, using "prothrombin time (PT)" instead of "nutritional status" (the following table), which finally formed a widely used modified Child–Pugh classification at present. According to the score, the liver function of patients can be divided into three levels: grade A: 5–6 points with small surgical risk; grade B: 7–9 points with moderate surgical risk; grade C: >10 points (including 10 points) with large surgical risk. Since its introduction, modified Child–Pugh classification has played an irreplaceable important role in surgical guidance for patients with liver cancer and liver cirrhosis.

4.3 Surgical Risk Assessment Methodology

The step of surgical risk evaluation is to sort and collect the existing disease conditions—evaluate the possibility of risk occurrence—and make risk ranking and grading.

4.3.1 Empirical Assessment

In the actual surgical work, most surgeons still use the more traditional method to assess the risk, including case analysis method, experience judgment method, expert survey method, etc., generally taking the previous personal or team experience as the basic disc, the author calls it the experience assessment method. As a traditional method of risk assessment, the empirical assessment method still has certain advantages, and the disadvantages are also more obvious. Judgment based on personal experience is simple and feasible, but due to the inherent limitations of personal knowledge, experience, and thinking, the risk evaluation within the scope of experience is often one-sided and appears to be helpless in the face of problems that have never occurred; learning from previous cases has better comprehensiveness, but due to the complex and individual case conditions, it is completely applicable; the expert survey method has greatly improved the breadth and depth of knowledge and experience, is scientific, but it is also susceptible to the subjective attitude of the expert team, and has a higher cost. In general, the traditional empirical assessment method still has its applicable soil at present, but in the context of further improvement of the scientific quality of surgeons in the future, it is historically inevitable that its application will be gradually reduced.

4.3.2 FMEA Method

The Failure Mode and Effects Analysis (FMEA) method originated in the American space industry in the 1960s and was gradually applied to medical risk evaluation in the 1990s. As a systematic and prospective analysis method, it mainly analyzes the possible effectiveness mode in the medical process and analyzes its possible consequences, so as to take necessary measures in advance, so as to inhibit the occurrence of risks. The core of FMEA method is to establish an interprofessional and multidisciplinary expert evaluation group to accurately describe the specific process of surgical diagnosis and treatment through extensive collection and collation of data, from which the failure mode, that is, the possible risk, and the corresponding risk factors and effects of further evaluation are determined. The key to FMEA is to calculate the Risk Priority Number (RPN), which is calculated as:

$$\text{RPN} = O \times D \times S.$$

where O (Occurrence) represents the probability of risk occurrence, D (Detection) represents the degree of detectability, and S (Severity) represents the severity. The above three can be scored according to the specific circumstances of each specialty. The RPN is the product of the three. The higher the score, the higher the risk. The FMEA method has been widely used abroad and has accumulated some experience, and domestic application is still in its infancy. The essence of FMEA is the evaluation of expert group and the comprehensive calculation of formula. The difference between FMEA and traditional expert discussion mode is that the process of risk evaluation is reasonably optimized, which is convenient for clinical realization of scientific management of risk evaluation process and the development of effective risk prevention plan.

4.3.3 Risk Matrix

Risk matrix is an effective risk evaluation tool, which was first proposed by the United States Air Force Electronics Center in the 1990s and popularized in the United States military weapon system development project. The purpose of risk evaluation is not to estimate the probability of risk or the degree of loss alone, but to assess the overall impact of risk factors on the results. The risk matrix comprehensively considers the impact of the probability of risk occurrence and the severity of adverse consequences. The risk matrix generally includes the risk occurrence probability, consequence severity, and risk level. The risk occurrence probability and consequence severity can be divided into different levels according to the specific circumstances of various specialties, while the risk level is determined by the former two, which can be generally divided into three to five levels. The author has tabulated surgical risks according to the above methods and classified surgical risk factors into four levels (Table 2.8).

The drawing of risk evaluation matrix is very simple from a technical point of view, and the visualization of the results also improves its feasibility and

Table 2.8 Surgical risk evaluation matrix

	Severity			
Probability of occurrence	Minor	Moderate	Serious	Death
Low	Low risk	Low risk	High risk	Very high risk
Lower	Low risk	Medium risk	High risk	Very high risk
Medium	Low risk	Medium risk	High risk	Very high risk
Higher	Medium risk	High risk	High risk	Very high risk
Well	Medium risk	High risk	Very high risk	Very high risk

convenience of application. The main difficulty lies in how to determine the probability of occurrence and severity of consequences of a certain risk factor. The surgical risks of different subspecialties are quite different. At present, the main method to solve the problem is still the investigation and review of experts in various fields. In the face of multiple evaluation experts or guidelines, the Borda ordinal method (a classical voting method, that is, the ranking voting system, and interested readers can consult the relevant books on their own) is usually used for importance ranking.

4.3.4 Risk Prediction Scoring Model

Although the aforementioned risk evaluation methods are relatively simple and easy, they are insufficient in the objectivity of the assessment based on the experience of individuals or teams. The risk prediction score model includes some simple and easy to measure risk factors into the statistical model, so as to predict the possibility and severity of the results. The same principle is also widely used in disease diagnosis or prognosis prediction. The rigorous risk prediction score model is usually based on large cohort study, requiring reasonable data volume and study design. The most commonly used statistical models are logistic models and Cox regression models, and logistic multivariate analysis is the most commonly used for surgical risk evaluation. Some of the more widely used risk prediction scoring models are listed for the reader in the next section.

Subjective risk evaluation is usually difficult to achieve very accurate, and more importantly, it is difficult to achieve accurate understanding of the specific impact of different risk factors on the results "ability" and the mutual influence between risk factors, which can easily cause inaccurate surgical risk evaluation results under the influence of multiple factors. The risk prediction score model overcomes the above difficulties from a statistical point of view, and it has a precise perception of the specific impact "ability" of each single factor in the multivariate analysis (at least for the included sample). It is worth mentioning that the first thing derived from sample statistics is the risk prediction model, rather than the risk prediction score. The risk scoring is a simplified version of the prediction model you build, and the weight of each variable can be used to calculate the score of each individual corresponding to the magnitude of the probability of occurrence. The risk prediction model accurately calculates the probability of a person's event according to the final basic risk and formula, and the calculation is complex. It is difficult for the mental arithmetic to calculate human brain and is inconvenient for clinical application. For the convenience of application, most of the risk prediction scoring models adjust the decimal number calculated by statistics and balance the accuracy with the practicability.

At present, there are a large number of risk prediction scoring models "made" in various academic papers, and only a small number have been widely recognized in clinical practice. Although it is safer to use widely recognized models, how to judge the quality of a risk prediction scoring model is still a valuable topic. Excellent prediction models should have good discrimination and calibration. Discrimination refers to the ability to distinguish between the level of risk in a group of people for an outcome, and it is usually related to the heterogeneity of risk factors (independent variables) included in the model. Discrimination is generally evaluated by the area under the ROC curve (AUC), and more than 0.75 is generally considered to be high discrimination. Calibration is a measure of the accuracy of the probability of an outcome event occurring in a certain individual in the future of the model, which reflects the degree of agreement between the risk predicted by the model and whether the risk actually occurs and is usually evaluated using the goodness of fit test (Hosmer–Lemeshow test). However, the use frequency of the above two indicators in the current literature is still worrying, so although the risk prediction score model is scientific, it still needs to use scientific methods to discover and evaluate, and the next step can be put into clinical application.

4.4 Common Risk Prediction Scoring Model

Risk scoring and risk prediction scoring models are important contents of surgical risk evaluation. Understanding, mastering, and flexibly applying various risk prediction scoring models can deepen the understanding of surgical risk evaluation. The author introduces two surgical risk prediction scores with representative significance and wide application. They have withstood the test of time, have been widely recognized, and adopt a more scientific statistical method, which has certain reference significance.

4.4.1 POSSUM Scoring System

At present, there are a variety of scoring systems for predicting the surgical risk of patients in clinical practice. Through these systems, health care providers can make predictive judgments about patient surgery in order to provide further treatment and services to patients. The POSSUM Score (Physiological and Operative Severity Score for the enumeration of Mortality and Morbidity), first established by the British scholar Copeland et al. in 1991, is one of the more influential and is a scoring system for predicting mortality and complication rates. It consists of two parts: physiological score and surgical severity score. The physiological score includes 12 indicators including patient age, cardiac signs, respiratory system, systolic blood pressure, pulse rate, Glasgow coma score, hemoglobin, white blood cells, serum urea, serum sodium, serum potassium, and electrocardiogram, which is an assessment of the general condition of the patient; the surgical severity score includes 6 indicators including surgical size, surgical urgency, intraoperative blood loss, degree of abdominal contamination, malignant degree of the tumor, and number of operations, which mainly assesses the surgical risks. After obtaining various scores, the mortality and complication rates of patients are calculated by special consensus, respectively.

POSSUM scoring system is originally a traditional method to predict the incidence of complications and mortality in patients after surgery. With the continuous improvement, more and more practices and studies have shown that compared with other surgical scoring systems, POSSUM scoring system is simpler in patient data collection, more objective results, and higher patient acceptance and understanding. Therefore, the POSSUM scoring system has been widely used in Europe and the USA and has become one of the important tools for perioperative risk evaluation.

Initially, POSSUM was mainly used in general surgery, vascular surgery, and cardiovascular surgery, and then Copeland et al. modified the POSSUM scoring system to design a scoring system suitable for orthopedics. Despite many advantages, the index analysis method applied by POSSUM scoring system is not generally accepted. In addition, many scholars believe that the score overestimates postoperative mortality, especially in low-risk groups; and the range of postoperative complications is large, with significant differences in complications between procedures, and prediction by the score is more general and less convincing.

After that, POSSUM scoring has been continuously improved, resulting in many improved versions with more application significance. Some scholars adopt the new statistical method under the premise of maintaining various indicators unchanged and obtain a logarithmic regression equation for more accurate prediction of postoperative mortality, which is called P-POSSUM (Portsmouth-POSSUM) scoring system; others use the Cr-POSSUM (Colorectal-POSSUM) scoring specially designed for colorectal surgery. This modified score simplifies the prediction indicators in POSSUM into 6 preoperative physiological indicators and 4 surgical invasiveness indicators, which is more concise and convenient, and the prediction accuracy is also higher; there are more M-POSSUM (Modified-POSSUM) scores more used in gastrointestinal surgery, and so on. Thus, the POSSUM scoring, a method for screening independent risk factors from multiple risk factors by multivariate analysis, has been widely recognized and is currently a typical case for risk evaluation.

4.4.2 Grading of Clavien-Dindo Surgical Complications

Surgical complications have become a “byproduct” that have plagued surgeons for many years due to the characteristics of surgery, that is, surgery itself can have traumatic or functional effects on the human body. It can even be said that surgical complications are the main surgical risks, and whoever controls surgical complications truly masters the essence of surgery—not just completing an operation, but keeping the damage to the patient to a minimum. Historically, however, mortality has been an important method for assessing surgical risk, and the classification and grading of postoperative complications have long been in an awkward situation that is not standardized, not consistent, or not complete. The entire surgical community lacks a set of scientifically standard methods or systems to evaluate postoperative complications, which seriously hinders the progress of surgical clinical research.

In 1992, Strasberg et al. classified postoperative complications of surgery into 4 categories (T92) according to the severity of various surgical complications, that is, the degree of negative prognosis of surgical treatment, and then developed a modified "accordion" severity grading system based on T92, including a simple grading (4 levels) and an extended grading (6 levels) system, and introduced a simple quantitative standard definition of terms and proposed a standard tabular reporting system. This allows for better grading of complications when studying major procedures that are very complex, such as esophagectomy or pancreatectomy with multiple serious complications, and the expanded complication grading system allows for a complete description of all complications. Since the development of a grading system to evaluate the severity of surgical complications (T92), investigators conducted a detailed study of 129 articles applying the complication grading system. It was found that these evaluation systems have a clear tendency to reduce the grading of surgical complications, to replace numerical grading with terms that have clear implications, and to present the severity of complications in different ways across grading systems that do not adequately meet the needs of surgical investigators.

In this context, Clavien–Dindo grading criteria were developed by Clavien and Dindo et al. in 2004 and modified Clavien-Dindo surgical complication grading criteria was developed in 2009. This standard, which has evolved over the years to provide a platform with excellent reliability and validity for the definition and grading of severity of postoperative complications, is now widely used and validated by hundreds of studies in many surgical fields.

Clavien–Dindo classification standardizes the grading of postoperative complications well, but in practical application, because of the "neglect" of less severe complications, it is possible that it does not represent the real overall postoperative morbidity. To summarize the overall incidence of postoperative complications, a composite index (CCI) was developed for all surgical procedures and their severity based on the widely established Clavien–Dindo classification. The essence of CCI is to determine the severity of a single complication using numerical simulation in the form of a questionnaire. This allowed for a summary of all postoperative complications of varying severity experienced by each patient, leading to an "original" CCI that reflected the overall incidence of postoperative complications. After further mathematical transformation, a final, easy-to-use CCI score is obtained, which effectively solves the above problems.

Although the Clavien–Dindo classification has not been proposed for a long time, it has been widely recognized by the surgical community, and its normative work on postoperative complications has a profound impact and is an important reference for surgical risk evaluation.

5 Surgical Risk Intervention

Surgical risk intervention is a chain process that follows the sequence of controlling the source of risk—reducing risk factors—reducing the loss caused by risk "occurrence, development, and outcome." First, controlling the source of risk represents a focus on the most fundamental cause of the risk, with the aim of prevention and control from the source of the risk. If standardized and proper preoperative evaluation is performed before surgery, preventive measures are given to patients with corresponding risks before surgery, such as jaundice reduction performed for patients with severe jaundice and preoperative implantation of artificial pacemakers in patients with arrhythmia. Second, we can also reduce losses by means of reducing risk factors. Such as emphasizing the management of disinfection procedures and regular safety inspection of intraoperative devices, and supervising the safety rules and regulations of medical wards and operating rooms. Surgical risk prevention refers to the process of taking measures for risk problems after risk identification and risk evaluation before the occurrence of risks. Surgical risk prevention is the core step in the surgical risk intervention system because it is really related to whether the possibility of eliminating or reducing the occurrence of adverse consequences before the risk occurs. Risk prevention is not only a technically difficult and detailed project, but also requires surgeons to take the courage subjectively and have the confidence of all staff to face and cope with risks after meticulous risk identification and objective risk evaluation. Finally, if after the above series of measures are taken, the risk sources and risk factors are not effectively controlled, and the risk accidents and adverse consequences still occur. At this time, the measures of "making up for the losses" are taken to reduce the losses, that is, surgical risk control. This section focuses on the rationale of surgical risk intervention in order to lay a theoretical foundation for the implementation process of risk intervention.

5.1 Concept of Risk Intervention

5.1.1 Development of Risk Prevention Concept

Many surgeons have a question in their hearts before and after seeing a patient or completing a surgical procedure: "Is there a problem with doing so, what are the consequences?" A small number of surgeons faced with such "uncertainty" chose to let the situation go, reassuring themselves that "there should be no problem." This is due to the fact that the concept of surgical prevention is not strong enough. In any surgical diagnosis and treatment process, its risks are objective and cannot be transferred due to the subjective will of the surgeon. As far as surgeons are concerned, only by facing the risks in thought and establishing the behavioral policy of active response, they can talk about the follow-up solutions to the risks. While surgeons can only learn and understand as much as possible about the objective laws of disease and risk, the emphasis on the concept of prevention is indeed something that every medical practitioner has the obligation and should be able to establish and achieve.

In the field of safety work, the famous Murphy's law and Hain rules are often mentioned [1].

Murphy's law is a psychological effect whose original sentence is "If there are two or more ways to do something, and one of them will lead to disaster, someone must make this choice." The fundamental content of any safety management, including medical safety field, is that "as long as there is a risk of causing accidents, no matter how small the probability is, accidents will always occur and will cause the greatest loss." The implication of Murphy's Law to the surgeon is that surgical risks that occur with a small probability should not be neglected. The low probability of a small event occurring during a patient's surgical visit paralyzes the surgeon, causing him or her to fail to take preventive interventions in a timely manner, instead leading to an increased probability of risk. It is considered that the fluke psychology of "small probability event will not occur" is the core cause of adverse consequences. As long as there are objective surgical risks, even if a small number of cases do not appear, as long as they continue to engage in diagnosis and treatment behaviors, they will certainly cause adverse consequences. Therefore, in response to surgical risks, no matter the probability of occurrence, it is necessary to strictly evaluate and take measures when necessary to control the possible adverse consequences in the embryonic stage.

Hain rules point out that behind each serious accident, there must be 29 minor accidents and 300 near misses and 1000 hidden dangers of accidents. Its implication lies mainly in two points. First, the occurrence of accidents is not accidental, but the inevitable result after various risk factors accumulate to certain achievements, that is, quantitative changes cause qualitative changes; second, no matter how perfect the technology and strict rules and regulations are, they cannot replace the staff's own quality and sense of responsibility in practical work. Hain rules remind every surgeon that accidents often have signs and that various hidden dangers and risk factors may induce serious consequences if they fail to attract enough attention. In addition, Hain rules place greater emphasis on human initiative, reminding surgeons that they should remain sensitive to all types of surgical risks and take measures in advance based on the principles and components of risk prevention.

Murphy's law points to the seriousness of the consequences and Hain rules emphasize the necessity of subjective prevention, which is a wake-up call for every surgeon. For all kinds of surgical risks, serious attitude should be taken at all times in order to achieve the best results.

5.1.2 Principles for Implementing Risk Control

Surgical risk control refers to that medical institutions or medical staff actively and consciously take measures after the occurrence of surgical risks to reduce the degree of adverse consequences and control injuries. Risk prevention is the active preventive action taken against a source of risk and risk factors to prevent or reduce the likelihood or severity of occurrence. Risk has already occurred when risk control is taken, and its fundamental purpose is to reduce the degree of injury and prevent further development of risk. Risk control cannot solve the cause of the risk, but it can effectively control the degree of damage caused by the risk and stop the subsequent risk cascade from occurring. The difference from risk prevention is that the effectiveness of risk control is after the occurrence of risk (Fig. 2.4).

The occurrence of surgical risks is often the trigger for medical disputes and accidents, therefore, in controlling surgical risks, in addition to responding calmly

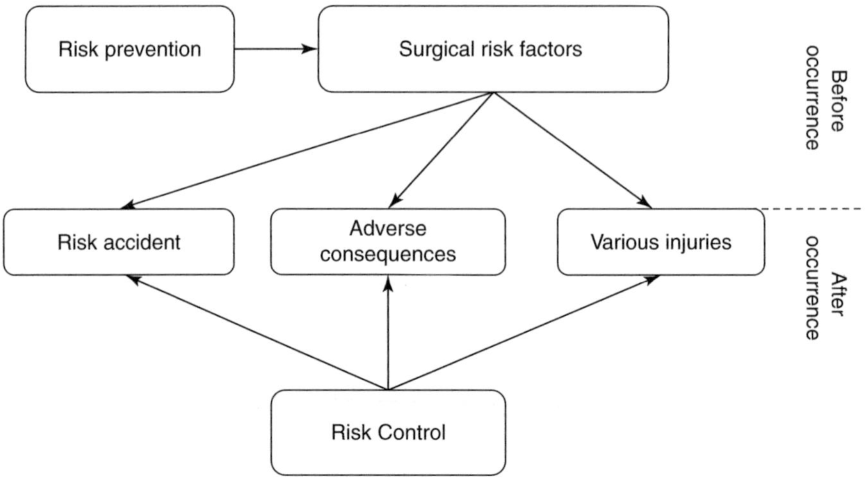

Fig. 2.4 Relationship between risk prevention and risk control

and dealing with them early in medical treatment, we should also pay attention to the correct view of the doctor–patient relationship, so as to be sensible, reasonable, and legal. When carrying out surgical risk control, medical staff shall pay attention to ensuring the safety of medical behaviors first. Surgery is a discipline with more invasive operations, more use of various instruments, and strong practicality, and it is often easy to cause accidents due to some mistakes. On the one hand, medical staff should comply with existing regulations or early warning plans, be realistic and proactive in dealing with the situation, and safety should be the first priority. We should strictly avoid solving problems beyond our ability without permission due to blind self-confidence or fear of responsibility and should evaluate risks calmly when they arise and call for the assistance of higher-level doctors or relevant departments for consultation if necessary to effectively maintain medical safety. Second, we pay attention to maintaining the doctor–patient relationship. Because the information of both doctors and patients in medical knowledge is completely asymmetric, and the patient himself/herself is ill, he/she reasonably seeks the doctor, which causes the actual inequality of the status of both doctors and patients. In terms of public opinion, patients are often considered to be vulnerable groups and are biased to some extent. As a medical staff, due to the existence of this objective situation, the rights and interests of patients and their families should be considered when dealing with risks. In practice, we should not rely on "talent" to be superior consciously, nor should we be afraid of being held responsible by the affected party and conceal the real situation. In case of any unexpected situation, we should communicate with the affected party in time. At the same time, attention should be paid to communication skills, focusing on ensuring patient safety and controlling surgical risks, and family members should not be deliberately induced to adopt excessive or negative treatment methods.

5.2 Principles of Surgical Risk Intervention

Surgical risk intervention is a highly purposeful task, and it is by establishing the goals of risk intervention that we can determine the direction and specific measures for risk prevention and evaluate the results.

5.2.1 Life Safety

Surgical risk prevention is a part of surgical risk intervention system, and its fundamental goal is to ensure the life safety of patients. For patients, the most serious consequence of surgical risks is loss of life. On the basis of ensuring life safety, the goal of surgical risk prevention is to make patients try not to have accidents in the diagnosis and treatment process and control the risks within an affordable range.

5.2.2 Risk Communication

Surgeons are obliged to make patients and their families aware of the existence of risks, rather than concealing risks, which is conducive to the affected side to improve risk awareness and actively cooperate with the implementation of risk prevention measures; however, they follow the principle of disease notification, once the risks occur, they can improve the acceptance of the affected side and avoid the embarrassing situation that both doctors and patients do not understand each other. However, at the same time, informing patients and their families of the existence of risks and their possible serious consequences will bring them a variety of concerns and fears and sometimes hinder their enthusiasm and cooperation in medical behavior. Therefore, the surgeons should make a scientific and objective statement on the surgical risks, do not deliberately amplify or reduce the impact of the risks, and provide reasonable advice from the perspective of the patient. Risk notification shall achieve the effect that patients can reduce their psychological burden and relieve their mental worries. The formation of a safe and reliable medical environment through risk communication is also an important goal of surgical risk prevention.

5.2.3 Reasonable Cost

After the first goal of ensuring the life safety of patients, it is also necessary to consider how to obtain the maximum risk prevention effect at the least cost, which requires that the risk prevention plan, scheme, and measure must be the most economical and reasonable before the risk accident actually occurs. The so-called reasonable cost, that is, to minimize unnecessary cost expenditure and waste, as far as possible to reduce the cost of risk prevention measures. However, objectively, cost reductions are often followed by an impact on the ultimate effectiveness of risk prevention, so how to balance cost and effectiveness becomes the key to achieving that goal.

Although there is a negative correlation between the two macroscopically, the details and know-how are not untraceable. For example, the length of time that a patient is admitted to the ICU after surgery and needs to be monitored in the ICU. If the patient has been admitted to ICU, the cost is high, and ICU monitoring may not reach relevant specialists at the specific professional level; if the patient is not admitted to ICU, the patient cannot receive strict and meticulous monitoring after operation, and his risk prevention may not be given. In fact, cost management is a decision-making problem for surgeons. Under the premise of regularization of medical norms, individualization of medical behavior based on experience is the key to balance the problem.

5.2.4 Risk Communication

In the process of risk intervention, risk communication refers to the process that medical staff and medical institutions communicate and transmit the information of risk-related factors (including risk causes, adverse consequences, handling methods, and other information).

In the traditional process of dealing with surgical risks, we pay more attention to the patient's condition, and it is easier to ignore the importance of internal communication among medical staff. This is because in the impression of many medical staff, risk intervention is still a more unfamiliar term and concept. When dealing with surgical risks, physicians and nurses are often more concerned with their own areas of concern and familiarity and issues while neglecting overall integrated planning. Therefore, in the early stage, department managers should establish an education system for risk intervention and provide knowledge and background education on risk intervention to each front-line medical care so that they understand the principles and methods of risk intervention. At the same time, each surgeon should have a collective awareness and strengthen the concept of honor and safety. In clinical work, because of the adverse effects caused by unclear explanation of the condition and weak risk awareness when handing over with succession, duty physicians, and nurses. This requires all medical staff to do a good job in risk exchange and connect the relay bar to ensure the safety of patients. In addition, it is emphasized that surgeons carry out comprehensive and detailed risk exchange with other physicians in the same department and consultants in other departments to achieve the best comprehensive diagnosis and treatment effect.

5.3 Specific Forms of Surgical Risk Intervention

After the surgeons have identified and evaluated the risks, and roughly determined the possibility of the risks and the severity of the consequences, they need to further analyze and consider the costs and effects of various risk intervention methods as the basis for risk decision-making. Any approach to risk intervention has its advantages and disadvantages and its inherent scope of use, and we need to be aware of the advantages and disadvantages of each approach and the circumstances of its use. In general, the modalities of surgical risk intervention mainly include risk prevention and risk control.

5.3.1 Risk Prevention

Risk prevention refers to the specific preventive measures adopted prior to occurrence of risk, with the goal of reducing the occurrence rate of surgical risks or damage degree of adverse consequences. Risk prevention is an active preventive measure. In order to achieve correct and reasonable risk prevention, it is necessary to analyze the risk factors, that is, risk prevention depends more on the risk identification, risk evaluation, and other early risk pre-control process. Risk prevention should follow the principle of targeting, which mainly deals with evaluated, evidence-based potential risks rather than imaginary, scientifically unproven, and unanalyzed conjectures.

Risk prevention measures are mainly effective before a risk occurs, that is, "beforehand" measures, which are designed to affect or interrupt the chain of risk occurrence and reduce the incidence or degree of injury of the risk. It mainly includes the following three aspects:

1. To influence the risk factors. For example, the evaluation of preoperative cardiopulmonary risk in patients with cardiovascular diseases reduces the possibility of intraoperative cardiovascular risk by changing the probability of overall potential cardiovascular risk in the surgical patient population. However, once intraoperative cardiovascular risk occurs, the consequences are usually serious and their severity will not be reduced due to preoperative evaluation.
2. To change the risk environment. For example, in hepatectomy, because the liver is a solid organ with an abundant blood supply, there is often more intraoperative bleeding. At this time, the risk factor is the physiological characteristics of the hepatic system, and we can change the blood pressure of the hepatic venous system by controlling the venous pressure and prevent the risk by changing the risk environment in which the liver is located.
3. To interrupt the downstream chain of risk factors. For example, for patients with splenomegaly secondary to cirrhosis-portal hypertension, causing secondary hypersplenism, splenectomy is used to avoid excessive cytopenias and prevent risk factors for cirrhosis from affecting the downstream. The preventive actions taken at this time do not address the source risk factors.

5.3.2 Risk Control

Another type of "afterwards" measure, risk control, is to address the reduction in the severity of an adverse consequence once a risk has occurred. For example, for patients with liver/kidney tumors and venous tumor thrombus, the tumor thrombus is easy to fall off during thrombectomy and causes fatal complications such as myocardial infarction and pulmonary embolism. At this time, the vein drains into the right atrium and is disposed into the filter to prevent emboli from entering the heart. It is a damage reduction measure, the filter cannot prevent emboli from falling off, but after emboli fall off, the filter can reduce its possibility of entering the heart. The so-called afterwards measures do not refer to post hoc remedies, but we have taken preventive measures in advance, but these measures can only work after the occurrence of risks.

Common risk control measures include rescue plan, emergency treatment plan, etc., that is, "afterwards" measures tend to be "plans," which is an "insurance" to cope with surgical risks, that is, to know the possible consequences in advance, and then deploy preventive measures. Intraoperative blood preparation and intraoperative consultation system of relevant departments are typical risk control measures. In addition, some risk interventions may function in both prevention and control. After the education and training of medical staff and the formulation of rules and regulations, the medical staff can not only actively prevent and reduce the incidence of risks from reducing human errors after the relevant knowledge learning and system standardization are carried out, while after the accident, the medical staff are also more familiar with the control measures, which can effectively improve the efficiency of risk control and reduce the severity of disease risks and the degree of losses.

In conclusion, surgical risk intervention is the most critical part of the surgical risk management system. Establishing the correct concept of prevention and mastering reasonable intervention measures are the keys to achieving surgical risk management. We need to pay attention to several aspects when performing surgical risk interventions: (1) Choosing interventions on the basis of cost and benefit. The intervention measures taken and the protection of patients shall be adapted to the severity of possible consequences. How to grasp the balance between cost (economic and labor costs of risk intervention) and benefit (patient safety) needs to be weighed according to the actual situation. Any risk intervention is costly, and in practice, it is easy to expend too much effort on the overprevention of low-risk accidents and instead ignore the high risk factors that really need to be prevented. (2) It cannot rely entirely on interventions. Risk interventions, whether based on machines or people, are inherently subject to the possibility of malfunction or failure. Therefore, for some serious consequences, multiple risk interventions should be used in combination according to the conditions, so as to reduce the risk of the disease as much as possible. (3) It cannot ignore the risks brought about by risk interventions. Some risk interventions reduce risk on the one hand and bring new risks on the other. Still using the example of splenectomy in a patient with hypersplenism, splenectomy is done to address the patient's risk of anemia, but splenectomy itself as a surgical procedure may cause a new series of risks. In summary, surgical risks are completely eliminated, but as surgeons, they should build confidence in coping with risks, strive to combine with the application of existing conditions, and continuously improve and optimize the intervention means to improve the prognosis of patients.

References

1. Cui JL, Wang YP. Murphy's law and Hein rules on medical safety. Med Philos B. 2012; 33(12):1–2.
2. Shao H, Xue MR. Unification, breakthrough and defect of the rules for the trial of liability dispute cases of medical damage — based on the analysis of the relevant provisions of the interpretation of the supreme people's court on several issues concerning the application of law in the trial of liability dispute cases of medical damage. Med Jurisdict. 2018;10(02):35–40.

Suggested Reading

Breasted JH. The Edwin smith surgical papyrus. The classics of medicine. Library. 1930;

Chen JM, Mao ZH. Risk factors and intervention measures of surgical site infection. Chin J Nosocomiol. 2012;(11):2302–4.

Chen XP, Qiu FZ, Wu ZD, et al. Causes, prevention and treatment of massive hemorrhage during hepatectomy. Chin J Surg. 2003;(03):15–7.

Gawande A. Two hundred years of surgery. N Engl J Med. 2012;366(18):1716–23.

Huang ZQ. Minimally invasive surgery and minimally invasive surgery - the main theme of surgery in the 21st century. Chin J Surg. 2002;1:9–12.

Huang ZQ. Traditional surgery and disappearing surgical tradition - historical outlook on development of surgery. J Digest Surg. 2005;(02):77–83.

Lister J. On a new method of treating compound fracture, abscess, etc., with observations on the conditions of suppuration. Lancet. 1867;89(2273):326–9.

Ma LB, Chai C, Cao N. Risk factors and preventive measures of surgical site infection. Chin J Bases Clin Gen Surg. 2014;(11):1444–7.

Mangram AJ, Horan TC, Pearson ML, et al. Guideline for prevention of surgical site infection. Am J Infect Control. 1999;27(2)

Margotta R, Li C. History of medicine; 2004.

Nutton V. Logic, learning, and experimental medicine. Science. 2002;295(5556):800–1.

Ren TG. Miraculous pivot of yellow emperor's classic of internal medicine people's military surgeon; 2006.

Su SH. History of open surgery. Citic Press; 2014.

Sun SM. Valuable prescriptions for emergency. China Medical and Technology Press; 2011.

Decision Making Process for Interveners 3

Rong Liu and Qu Liu

Abstract

This chapter focuses on the clinical decision-making of interveners. First, it describes the classification, characteristics, and influencing factors of clinical decision-making. Then, the process of clinical thinking and the thinking methods in clinical decision-making are described in detail. On the basis of this, it puts forward four suggestions on how to develop clinical thinking. Clinical decision-making must be evidence-based and should not be limited by clinical subspecialties, so this chapter further introduces the application of evidence-based medicine and MDT model in clinical decision-making.

1 Clinical Decision-Making

Decision-making is omnipresent in our lives, and as long as there is a choice, it involves the problem of decision-making. In our lives and work, we often encounter the "donkey effect" proposed by the French philosopher Buridan. A donkey stood hesitant between two piles of hay of exactly the same quantity, quality, and distance. Because the donkey could not distinguish between the advantages and disadvantages of two piles of hay, helpless stood in place and finally starved to death alive. The difficulty this donkey encountered in decision-making was Buridan "donkey effect." As the saying goes: "You can't have both the fish and the bear's paw." Everyone often faces a variety of decisions in life, and how to choose is extremely important for the success of things and even the success or failure of life. In order to obtain the best results, people often weigh and deliberate in their choices. But in

R. Liu (✉) · Q. Liu
Faculty of Hepato-pancreato-biliary Surgery, Chinese PLA General Hospital, Beijing, China
e-mail: liurong301@128.com

R. Liu (ed.), *Clinical Decision Making for Improving Prognosis*,
https://doi.org/10.1007/978-981-19-2952-6_3

many cases, the opportunity is fleeting and requires us to make decisions immediately and quickly. If we hesitate, we will get nothing.

The object of medicine is people, and intervention providers, including doctors, make various decisions every day, which are often related to patient health or even life safety. For example, what laboratory tests are scheduled? What drug should be used? Is surgery required? When to choose which surgical option? The treatment of postoperative critical illness and the choice of clinical supportive treatment. So, what is the best clinical decision? Different intervention providers may make completely different decisions for the same patient with the same clinical data. Making the right decisions is the only way to have success and hope for life. If the decision is wrong, no matter how superb the technology will not achieve satisfactory results. Therefore, it is particularly important how intervention providers make prompt and accurate clinical decisions.

1.1 Definitions

Clinical decision-making is based on the basic principles of medicine, according to the clinical experience of intervention providers, including doctors, in combination with the specific circumstances of patients, after fully assessing the risks and benefits of different options, to make choices and implement the relevant issues in the treatment process of diseases. The clinical decision-making of all intervention providers needs to be taken seriously by us, and how to guide them to make reasonable and effective clinical decisions requires further research and attention.

1.2 Classification

Clinical decision-making covers the whole process from diagnosis to treatment, including not only strategic, that is, the overall medical treatment principles, but also tactical decision-making, according to specific patients and specific circumstances, to take specific decisions. In general, clinical decisions are divided into the following three categories according to timeliness:

1. Flexible decision-making: This decision has a certain flexibility in the time limit and can be consulted with information or consulted with teachers and colleagues before making a decision. Flexible decision-making mainly covers general decisions that occur in the ward, including predicting potential risks and formulating routine treatment and surgical plans.
2. Time-limited decision-making: This decision requires judgment and selection within a limited period of time. It usually occurs in outpatient work, giving a diagnosis to patients who visit the clinic and treating them in a timely manner. While such decisions do not involve a life-and-death test, do not require an immediate decision and can have time to consider, they should also be made as soon as possible in most cases.

3. Urgent decision-making: Urgent decision-making is the decision to make a prompt judgment and choice and can directly affect the treatment and prognosis of patients. For example, in the emergency department, intervention providers often encounter patients with car accidents and multiple systemic injuries, which are very critical, and patients are often in a state of shock and dyspnea, which trauma is the most life-threatening for patients? What problems should be solved first to maximize life saving and reduce trauma? In addition, in complex surgical procedures requiring speed, courage, and skills, when critical risks come, intervention providers need to be calm, unfrightened, and tacit to cooperate, and find key points to control risks based on the usual accumulation and reserve of clinical experience and surgical skills in order to save the danger. At this time, decision-making is often directly related to the prognosis and life safety of patients, with the highest requirements for intervention providers, and only long-term clinical training and accumulation, coupled with strong and stable psychological quality, rapid and correct decision-making can be made.

1.3 Characteristics of Clinical Decision-Making

1.3.1 Integrity

Clinical decision-making is not only limited to the treatment itself, but also includes the diagnosis of diseases, preoperative evaluation, timing of surgery, selection of surgical methods, control of intraoperative risks, intervention and evaluation and treatment of postoperative complications. Therefore, a holistic view is needed for clinical decision-making, and patients must not be fragmented into isolated organs, seeing only the trees but not the forest. It is necessary not only to pay attention to the functional recovery of diseased organs and the success of treatment, but also to the rehabilitation of the patient's overall function. Otherwise, the surgical skills are no longer skillful, which is only the "cutter" of the operation. In some cases, there will be the extreme phenomenon that although the tumor is removed, the patient has lost his vital signs during the surgery. Therefore, clinical decision-making should have a holistic view, pay attention to the integrity of the intervention process, run all aspects of diagnosis and treatment into the clinical decision-making system, and also pay attention to the integrity of the patient's physiological function. In addition to paying attention to the mechanism and function of injured organs, pay attention to the stability of vital signs and the synergy of multiple organ functions, so as to ensure the safety and rapid recovery of patients.

1.3.2 Risk

Clinical decision-making is related to the functional recovery and even life safety of patients, and its risk runs through the process of medical intervention. The risks are: (1) First, they come from the patients. There are many uncertainties in patients themselves, especially in elderly and critically ill patients. Not only is the development and outcome of the disease difficult to foresee and control in clinical practice, but also the response of patients to treatment is not the same, and even unpredictable serious complications may occur. These require close observation and timely response by intervention providers, without the slightest relaxation. It is impossible to have exactly the same patient in the world and there is no static clinical decision; (2) Even if the risk is known, the chance of occurrence is uncertain. Clinically, patients' families often ask about the incidence of risk. In fact, the incidence of risk is statistically significant in clinical research and treatment for a large sample of patients. However, for a single patient, once the risk occurs, it is 100%. Even the risk with a very small incidence often occurs due to the negligence of the intervention provider or the mutation of the condition, and unprepared phenomena often occur if the intervention providers do not do a good job of prediction and prevention; (3) The medical treatment itself is risky, and both drug intervention and surgical treatment are double-edged sword, with the possibility of iatrogenic injury and various adverse reactions. Moreover, the current medical understanding of many diseases and their occurrence mechanism are not clear, the understanding of the side effects of drugs and intervention treatment is not comprehensive, and effective prevention of all conditions cannot be achieved; (4) The medical technology level itself in different regions has great limitations and imbalance, and the knowledge, technology, thinking, and courage of intervention providers vary widely, which has a great impact on the final results of treatment, so intervention providers themselves are the key links affecting the risk of decision-making; (5) There are various differences in the management within hospitals and the synergy between professional teams, which will affect the implementation of clinical decisions and the therapeutic effect of patients.

1.3.3 Sociality

Clinical decision-making is not only a scientific problem, but also a social problem, which requires all-round thinking, not only involving academic problems, but also emphasizing the social environment and the non-technical cultivation of intervention providers. Many times medical disputes are caused by the lack of communication between intervention providers such as doctors and nurses and patients and their families, rather than simply due to medical technical problems. In order to improve the clinical decision-making ability, in addition to improving the medical technology level, the intervention providers should pay more attention to the psychological factors and social situation of patients, and emphasize the comprehensive improvement of psychological comfort, crisis assessment and communication and coordination ability. In clinical practice, it is necessary to closely link clinical decision-making with the system of knowledge, experience, skills, psychology, determination, coordination, communication and other conditions in order to cultivate optimized clinical decision-making ideas, methods, and skills.

1.4 Influencing Factors

Clinical decision-making includes many aspects from diagnosis to treatment, including the problem of selecting examination items and proposing hypothesis diagnosis, but also the problem of selecting treatment timing and treatment options. The factors affecting clinical decision-making exist in all aspects of the above, and each factor has uncertainty. Making the right decision among these many uncertainties is not easy. Clinical decision-making is the choice and measure taken by intervention providers for practical problems often faced in clinical practice, especially in the face of multiple choices or urgent situations requiring immediate decision, how to select the most correct method is a problem that we should focus on. In clinical practice, intervention providers often make decisions based on their clinical experience and ability; however, experience and ability often have personal limitations, and conformity psychology, celebrity effect, and even compassion for patients in decision-making can affect intervention providers' decision choices.

The first is the progress and development of medicine. With the rapid development of Internet medical information and artificial intelligence technology, the continuous maturity of molecular targeting and cancer immunotherapy, and the continuous emergence of high-tech represented by surgical robots, the continuous update of these medical technologies and concepts has made the optional diagnostic and therapeutic means more and more abundant and to make appropriate clinical decisions requires that intervention providers can keep pace with the times and walk at the forefront of the professional field at all times. Only by understanding and mastering the latest medical achievements, the best therapeutic means can be selected. For example, liver cancer is known as the "king of cancer", the initial treatment of liver cancer only surgical resection of this treatment, with the development of medical technology and the progress of concept, there will be anhydrous alcohol injection, radiofrequency ablation, interventional therapy and other minimally invasive treatment. At present, with the research progress of gene and immunotherapy targets, the application of targeted drugs and immune checkpoint inhibitors provides a variety of therapeutic means for the treatment of liver cancer, greatly improving the therapeutic effect of liver cancer. In terms of surgical methods alone, it has also developed from the initial laparotomy with great trauma to minimally invasive laparoscopy or even robotic minimally invasive surgery; from local resection to anatomical resection to the current three-dimensional reconstruction and fluorescence-guided hepatectomy; a variety of surgical methods such as anterior approach hepatectomy, phased hepatectomy combined with liver segmentation and portal vein ligation have also been derived, which greatly improves the accuracy of surgery, expands the indications, and reduces the trauma of patients. Therefore, only by comprehensively grasping the field of expertise and research progress represented by physicians, intervention providers can make the most accurate and reasonable clinical decisions according to different disease stages and the actual situation of patients.

The second is the own ability level. Medicine is a high-risk industry and a practical discipline. Intervention providers are required to experience numerous clinical practices over a long period of time, laying a solid foundation for their own growth and accumulation. However, each intervention provider has different knowledge, experiences, and medical platforms, which makes their clinical experience, academic level, and psychological quality vary widely, and these may affect the choice of clinical decision-making. The author's own ability not only refers to the theoretical knowledge and clinical experience and ability of medicine, but also includes his own professional level and accumulated clinical experience. He needs to be good at using the evidence of evidence-based medicine, learning experience from multidisciplinary consultation, using the advanced results brought about by new technologies such as artificial intelligence, and comprehensively improve the ability to make rapid and accurate clinical decisions in the face of clinical problems.

Third, coordinate the problem of management level. In the actual diagnosis and treatment process, the author often finds that there will be deviations in the judgment of the condition, the choice of decision-making, and the effect of treatment between doctors at the same level in the same department. In this case, the influencing factors of clinical decision-making may not only be limited to medical level and clinical experience, but also affect the results of decision-making and the outcome of treatment. Now disease treatment is often not limited to a single discipline, but requires multi-departmental and multi-professional coordination, requires the cooperation of multiple intervention providers, and the differences in coordination and management levels can be reflected at this time. Doctors with high coordination and management level can timely dispatch and communicate various departments after discovering problems and integrate multiple disciplines into a joint force to achieve the best therapeutic effect. The improvement of coordination management level is not innate and not achieved overnight, and it needs to be planned in advance and continuously accumulated to exercise multidisciplinary communication and coordination management ability in each practice of clinical treatment.

1.5 Significance

In today's era of knowledge economy, knowledge is money and decision-making is life. The nature of the intervention provider's work determines the need to face clinical decision-making at all times, and in a successful case, 75% lies in clinical decision-making and 25% is experience and skills. The correctness of clinical decision-making is related to the therapeutic effect of patients, determines the prognosis and outcome of patients, and even directly relates to the life and death of patients. At the same time, clinical decision-making is also very important for the growth of intervention providers. An accurate and effective clinical decision-making is a test for intervention providers and an embodiment of medical knowledge, experience, clinical thinking, and judgment ability. Improving clinical decision-making ability is not only the requirement for each intervention provider to improve professional quality, but also the inevitable requirement to comply with the development of the times and medical progress, and it is also an essential link in establishing a mutual trust doctor–patient relationship and creating a harmonious medical environment. Therefore, clinical decision-making, as the product of the combination of medical theory and practice, has a positive role in improving the accuracy and effectiveness of clinical interventions and reducing unnecessary social cost consumption.

2 Development of Clinical Thinking

In the complex clinical work, the patient's condition changes rapidly, the examination means are various, and the treatment methods are changing rapidly. Each intervention provider is intentionally or unintentionally applying the thinking method to solve the clinical problems in the actual work. Intervention providers should not only have solid basic theory, but also have scientific clinical thinking, and superb treatment techniques, in order to better deal with clinical intractable diseases. This chapter focuses on how to cultivate clinical thinking in order to improve the diagnosis and treatment of intervention providers.

2.1 Concept

Thinking refers to the process of obtaining rational cognition through abstraction, induction, deduction, analysis, and synthesis. Clinical thinking is a series of cognitive processes such as judgment, analysis, reasoning, and treatment of diseases by the intervention provider using existing basic theories and clinical experience. Clinical thinking plays a pivotal and central role in the entire healthcare process. Clinical thinking is characterized by strict timeliness, patient specificity, and dynamic course of the disease.

Careful and reasonable clinical thinking can make the disease get timely diagnosis and achieve satisfactory therapeutic effect, which plays an extremely important role in the judgment of disease risk and its prognosis, the selection of surgical timing and methods, and the prevention of surgical complications. Under the condition of similar objective conditions and knowledge level, the intervention providers with high level of clinical thinking can usually diagnose the diseases that are not seen by others or adopt the treatment methods unexpected by others, so that the difficult cases can be timely and accurately diagnosed and treated. Intervention providers with low clinical thinking skills, however, are at risk for cognitive biases that can lead to misdiagnosis, underdiagnosis, and missed treatments, thereby delaying the condition and causing patients to bear undue losses. Therefore, only by focusing on strengthening the training of clinical thinking methods, intervention providers can adopt correct understanding methods, make reasonable judgment and treatment, and make patients achieve the best therapeutic effect in the process of clinical diagnosis and treatment.

2.2 Process of Clinical Thinking

Clinical thinking mainly includes longitudinal thinking and horizontal thinking. Longitudinal thinking runs through the whole process of diagnosis and treatment regimen, including disease diagnosis, grasping surgical indications, making surgical plan, implementing surgical plan and postoperative treatment. Horizontal thinking is a horizontal extension of each step, such as differential diagnosis, selection of multiple treatment options, intraoperative decision-making, etc. The clinical thinking of the intervention provider is actually a process in which longitudinal and horizontal thinking intersect.

What the intervention provider sees just one aspect of the disease when seeing the patient. In the case of incomplete clinical data, it is inevitable that making diagnostic and therapeutic opinions will be one-sided. Therefore, it is also necessary to continuously collect new clinical data, improve the necessary examinations, observe the symptoms and signs, disease development and treatment response, so as to verify or revise the diagnosis and improve the treatment regimen. Through the process of rediagnosis and retreatment, until the final diagnosis is obtained and the final treatment regimen is determined.

2.2.1 Thinking Methods in Diagnostic Decision-Making

Diagnosis is the process of data collection, investigation, and study of patients. Judgment is the result of analysis and induction, deduction, and inference of the collected data. Clinical thinking begins with diagnosis, and in the process of making a diagnosis, intervention providers perform targeted physical examinations and auxiliary examinations based on clinical data of differential significance, so as to provide a basis for further definitive diagnosis.

Investigation and Collection of Clinical Data

The basis for establishing a primary diagnosis for a patient begins with the collection of data. The investigation and collection of clinical data mainly include medical history collection, physical examination, laboratory tests, and imaging examination. The medical history should be taken in as comprehensive and detailed as possible to grasp the process of disease development and evolution, and attention needs to be paid to meaningful clinical symptoms and negative symptoms of differential significance to provide ideas and clues for further examination. After taking the medical history, the intervention provider has formed a preliminary impression of the disease, guided by these impressions, and then a comprehensive physical examination is performed on the patient, focusing on the examination of the physical evidence of diagnostic and differential diagnostic significance, and purposefully selecting laboratory tests and imaging tests with high sensitivity and specificity. In today's rapidly changing auxiliary examinations, the optimization principle should be implemented according to the characteristics of different diseases and the specific circumstances of patients, and the order and combination of examinations should be selected.

Collation and Analysis of Clinical Data

In the face of intricate clinical data, intervention providers need to sort out, analyze, and summarize the data. There are both problems of professional ability and problems of thinking methods. When analyzing and organizing the data, the subjective initiative of the intervention provider should be fully utilized, and the professional knowledge should be applied to make a comprehensive analysis of the obtained materials through the clinical thinking of removing the crude, removing the false and keeping the true, from the surface to the inside, and from there to the other.

In the collation and analysis of clinical data, intervention providers should do the following: (1) Grasp the main contradictions and solve the most important current disease problems of patients. Patients may suffer from a variety of diseases at the same time when seeking medical treatment, but what needs to be solved this time must be the most urgent and troublesome problem for patients, so it is particularly important to grasp the main contradiction when analyzing the data. (2) In the complex clinical data, it is necessary to sort out the relationship between clinical symptoms, physical examination, and auxiliary examination in order to further speculate the possible location, nature, and etiology of the lesion and lay the foundation for definitive diagnosis. (3) In reality, there are many confounding factors that can affect the accuracy of examination data, which requires the intervention provider to carefully review and verify clinically suspicious materials to remove doubts and identify authenticity.

Formation of Hypothetical Diagnosis

After the investigation and collection, analysis and collation of clinical data, using the accumulated knowledge theory and clinical experience, the thinking process of analogy, induction, analysis, reasoning, deduction, etc. is carried out, and one or several hypothetical diagnoses are proposed, so as to form a preliminary diagnosis. There are three main thinking methods to form hypothetical diagnosis:

1. Exclusion diagnostic method. When a group of diseases with similar clinical manifestations occurs, they are compared with each other and excluded one by one to narrow the scope of differential diagnosis. When proposing a group of diseases to be identified, priority should be given to common and multiple diseases and closely related to reality. Specific analysis of specific problems should be performed. And all possible diseases should be included as much as possible to prevent misdiagnosis caused by omission. For example, patients with upper gastrointestinal bleeding need to match the characteristics of the disease with five common diseases, such as gastroduodenal ulcer bleeding, esophageal variceal bleeding, tumor bleeding, stress ulcer, and biliary tract bleeding, and those who meet the requirements are the preliminary diagnosis.
2. Reasoning diagnostic method. We should grasp a major symptom or sign in the clinical manifestation and gradually think deeply according to the clinical characteristics and mechanism of the disease, and finally make a reasonable diagnosis. For example, for patients with acute abdomen, we should grasp the main symptoms of abdominal pain, according to its pathogenesis and physiological characteristics, combined with the location, nature, degree, radiological characteristics, symptoms of abdominal pain, etc., follow the vine to get the melon and finally determine the root cause of abdominal pain.
3. Comprehensive diagnostic method. Comprehensive use of exclusion method and reasoning method facilitates the selection of further targeted tests and improves the accuracy of diagnosis through the comprehensive analysis of interrelated symptoms, signs, and test results. For specific patients, intervention providers

need to adapt to local conditions when using diagnostic thinking, flexibly use exclusion method, reasoning method, and comprehensive method, and integrate longitudinal thinking and horizontal thinking.

In clinical practice we need to pay attention to: (1) When making a hypothetical diagnosis, we should pay attention to the judgment made at the first consultation. The thinking of the first consultation determines the subsequent examination and treatment means, and any deviation may affect the direction of diagnosis and treatment. (2) Intervention providers attending the clinic should also not blindly rely on the diagnosis made at the first visit, because the judgment made in the outpatient and emergency department in a short period of time may be biased and need to be treated rationally. (3) In order to improve the accuracy of diagnosis, multiple consecutive examinations can be performed, or several examination methods can be used simultaneously or sequentially to improve the sensitivity and specificity of diagnosis. (4) Routine examination methods may have one or other shortcomings. With the development of medicine, new auxiliary examination methods will continue to appear. Intervention providers should continuously learn new diagnostic methods to enrich the diagnostic means and improve the diagnostic coincidence rate.

Validation of Hypothetical Diagnosis

After the hypothetical diagnosis is proposed, the intervention provider needs to further verify the hypothesis through examination, treatment, and observation, so as to draw a conclusion supporting or denying the original diagnosis. In clinical work, to make the correct diagnosis and treatment decisions, it is important to first recognize the hypothetical nature of the diagnosis and almost all clinical diagnoses are initially hypothetical. Second, for each examination and analysis by the intervention provider, only one cross-section at a certain stage in the disease process can be seen, and multiple cross-sections often have to be synthesized in order to understand the complete face of the disease. Moreover, the condition is continuously developing and changing, and clinical thinking is also a continuously progressive process. This requires looking at hypothetical diagnosis with a developmental perspective, observing the trend of disease development, observing the treatment response under the guidance of hypothetical diagnosis, continuously verifying and revising hypotheses, and timely revising treatment options.

Especially in the diagnosis and treatment of acute and severe diseases, under the pressure of severe condition and urgent time, the intervention provider needs to make a preliminary diagnosis immediately after a simple interview and treatment and take corresponding examination and treatment. In the process of examination and treatment, the hypothetical diagnosis is verified, and the next examination and treatment regimen is proposed. Therefore, sometimes the original diagnosis may be partially or completely modified. On the one hand, intervention providers need to continuously enrich their own knowledge and theoretical level, and on the other hand, they should study and summarize the causes of misdiagnosis, enrich clinical experience, and strive to improve the diagnostic level.

2.2.2 Thinking Method in Treatment Decision-Making

Once the diagnosis is confirmed, further treatment regimens need to be developed as soon as possible. If surgical treatment is required, there are problems in choosing the timing of surgery, surgical approach, intraoperative decision-making, postoperative management, and response to unexpected events. When formulating treatment decisions, intervention providers should choose among various treatment options and make reasonable treatment decisions by judging the risks and benefits in treatment and applying standardized and meticulous clinical thinking methods.

Development of Treatment Regimen

Intervention providers need to develop a practical and optimal treatment regimen for each patient, so it should vary from person to person and from disease to disease. Compared with the diagnostic process, the presence of more uncertain factors in treatment requires extensive clinical experience, social experience, and thinking ability. When formulating the treatment regimen, the intervention provider must consider many aspects, such as the complications of the disease, treatment complications, the physical condition of the patient, social and psychological conditions (family, marriage, economy, culture, personality, occupation, living habits and religious beliefs, etc.), current medical conditions and the experience and technical level of medical staff.

Treatment modalities can be mainly divided into non-surgical and surgical treatment. There are many types of non-surgical treatment, such as drug therapy, radiotherapy, physical therapy, etc., and surgical treatment includes open therapy and minimally invasive therapy. Each treatment has its clear indications and contraindications, but the two are not separated, but interrelated, and the therapeutic benefit can be maximized if it can be used with appropriate combination. For example, perioperative treatment is essentially part of non-surgical treatment, which can create conditions for surgical treatment and ensure smooth postoperative recovery. After surgical resection of the lesion by malignant tumors, it creates conditions for further comprehensive treatment such as chemoradiotherapy.

Therefore, how to select and arrange the order of multiple treatment methods can not only exert the greatest advantages of each treatment, but also avoid or reduce its adverse reactions, all of which require repeated comparison by intervention providers, weighing the advantages and disadvantages of various methods, and selecting the best method or optimal combination.

Decision-Making Thinking in the Perioperative Period

Preoperative Preparation

Surgery is one of the most important links in surgical decision-making. The difficulty and risk of surgery are fully estimated before the surgery, and the surgery is carefully planned, and a variety of possible plans are made according to the possible situations during the surgery, so as to perform devise strategies within a command tent during the surgery. Even emergency surgery should be performed after necessary preoperative preparation and must not be rashly performed.

The main problems facing preoperative preparation are the grasp of surgical indications as well as the assessment of the patient's ability to tolerate the procedure. This requires a clear preoperative diagnosis and an adequate estimation of the severity of the disease. When all clinical data are unable to make a clear diagnosis, laparotomy or laparoscopic exploration can also be used as a clear diagnosis method. In addition, it is necessary to have a sufficient understanding of the patient's general condition. Different surgeries have different requirements on the patient's tolerance ability, so in addition to a comprehensive physical examination and auxiliary examinations before surgery, targeted examinations should be conducted according to the special requirements of different surgeries on organ function in order to correctly assess the patient's tolerance ability for surgery. For patients with poor tolerance, in addition to general preoperative preparation, reasonable methods should also be used to improve the patient's tolerance to surgery. If patients with cirrhosis undergo hemihepatectomy or extended hemihepatectomy, liver functional reserve should be fully estimated, and portal vein branch embolization and ALPPS surgery can be performed if necessary to improve the function of preserving liver tissue. Effective preoperative correction of imbalances in water and electrolyte metabolism and acid–base balance in patients with tumors and obstructive jaundice can significantly improve the patient's ability to tolerate surgery. In addition, heart disease, hypertension, respiratory dysfunction, liver and kidney disease, diabetes, low immune system function and malnutrition and other diseases will seriously reduce the surgical tolerance of patients and should be corrected within the allowable range to improve the surgical tolerance.

The timing of surgery depends on the severity of the disease itself, the rate of progression, and the presence of life-threatening complications and according to this, surgery can generally be divided into elective surgery, limited surgery, and emergency surgery. If the liver malignancy is originally a limited surgery, emergency treatment is required if it is associated with rupture and bleeding of the tumor, which may lead to shock and tumor dissemination in patients.

Intraoperative Decision-Making

Intraoperative decision-making mainly includes intraoperative diagnosis, judgment of resectability, selection of surgical methods, and treatment of intraoperative critical conditions. During the operation, it is necessary to conduct a comprehensive exploration of the surgical area, focus on the examination of diseased organs, and perform rapid frozen pathological examination when necessary to confirm or correct the diagnosis. With the further understanding of the severity and extent of the disease, which surgical plan should be used should be comprehensively considered according to the patient's disease, the technical level of the surgeon, and the conditions of the device and equipment. The choice of surgical methods should follow the principle of the greatest benefit to patients, pay attention to the unity of radicality and safety, and the safety of patients is always ranked first in any case. The surgical operation should be strictly grasped to avoid the phenomenon of surgery for the purpose of surgery and reduce the blindness and arbitrariness of treatment. It is also necessary to consider the cost–benefit ratio as well as the progress of new theories and technologies to provide the basis for surgical intervention providers to make the optimal decision.

For various inevitable emergencies that may occur during surgery, such as massive hemorrhage, organ injury, etc., the surgical intervention provider should have sufficient psychological and technical preparation, and operations such as clamping in panic and hemostasis must not occur. Intraoperative iatrogenic injury often brings more serious trauma to the patient. Surgical intervention providers should plan ahead for possible unexpected risks and treatment plans, take precautionary measures, and pay attention to the cultivation of emergency response ability in general in order to cope with emergencies when they occur and turn them into success.

Postoperative Treatment

The purpose of postoperative treatment is to make the patients recover their physiological function as soon as possible, prevent and timely treat various postoperative complications, and promote the patients to recover as soon as possible. It should be fully recognized that surgery is an invasive procedure, and any surgical treatment can cause physical and psychological burden and trauma to patients. The intervention provider should be people-oriented, have a deep understanding of the pathophysiological changes that may be caused by surgery, pay attention to maintaining important organ function, water electrolyte, and acid–base balance, and develop a plan and regimen for medication on this basis. For postoperative complications, on the one hand, preventive measures should be implemented as early as possible to pinch the source of complications in advance and prevent problems before they occur; on the other hand, attention should be paid to observation, early diagnosis and treatment should be given at the early stage of complications through careful clinical observation to prevent the spread and further deterioration of complications and control the damage in the minimum range; on the other hand, the causes should be found from preoperative preparation, intraoperative operation, and postoperative management, self-criticism method should be used to summarize the lessons learned, improve clinical experience and clinical thinking, achieve risk pre-control, reduce the incidence of complications, and improve the prognosis of patients.

2.3 How to Cultivate Clinical Thinking

2.3.1 Diligent in Summing up

Clinical thinking ability will inevitably be improved in long-term clinical practice, but there is a fundamental difference between conscious improvement and natural improvement. "To learn without thinking is confusing, to think without learning is dangerous," and it is often encountered in clinical practice that surgical intervention providers with similar seniority often have different gains and improvements when their practice opportunities are similar, and the difference is mainly whether they are good at thinking and summarizing. Thinking refers to the thinking activities such as judgment, analysis, and reasoning for a certain phenomenon and is a purposeful active exploration. Through thinking, the essence of things can be understood through surface phenomena. In the process of clinical thinking, we should encourage and advocate early preparation and active thinking. Surgical intervention providers need to read films when diagnosing and treating patients, and good reading ability can not only quickly find clues to a definite diagnosis from imaging data, but also develop surgical plans in advance, which is a key link in the clinical thinking and skills of surgical intervention providers. And how to improve reading ability? This requires the intervention provider to think diligently, not only learn and summarize from the imaging report, but also need the anatomy in the comparison, and then repeatedly read and summarize after surgery. With the continuous increase of practice, observation, and thinking, the clinical thinking ability will be naturally improved.

Active thinking also lies in timely summary, as an intervention provider, his/her own continuous reflection and summary is also one of the most effective ways to improve clinical thinking ability. Because most of the common acute abdominal diseases in clinical practice have similar symptoms, variable conditions and urgent treatment, misdiagnosis and mistreatment often occur. When this situation is encountered, it is necessary to timely summarize the experience and lessons, summarize the experience of definite diagnosis and timely treatment in the complex disease data, and exercise the clinical thinking in practice. Academician Wu Mengchao, the father of hepatobiliary surgery in China, often said that "do, speak and write" is actually to summarize the phenomena observed in clinical practice and accumulated experience, summarize the regular theoretical understanding, and carry forward its dissemination through conference speeches and paper publication, which is not only to improve the individual clinical thinking ability, but also to trigger the thinking and accumulation of others, and finally drive the common progress in the relevant professional fields.

2.3.2 Focus on Practice

Clinical medicine is a highly practical and applied science, clinical thinking must be cultivated and improved in practice and exercises, not just based on book knowledge, behind closed doors, and dogmatic solutions to practical clinical problems. With the rapid development of medical science and technology, such as color Doppler ultrasound, CT, magnetic resonance, gastrointestinal endoscopy, PET-CT, and a series of advanced diagnosis and treatment methods applied in clinical practice, the cognitive ability of intervention providers for the disease has been greatly enriched and enhanced, resulting in that relatively some intervention providers only pay attention to the test data and test report and never carefully observe the symptoms and signs of patients. This approach of seeing the trees but not the forest will only confine the clinical thinking of the intervention provider and lead to misdiagnosis when the test results are interfered with by multiple factors or contradict each other. Therefore, in clinical practice, any modern examination method is only an extension of the intervention provider's senses and cannot replace the intervention provider's thinking, and the intervention provider cannot blindly rely on advanced examination means and ignore the overall and comprehensive grasp of the condition. When selecting the examination and treatment means, the intervention provider should also go deep into the patients, collect the first-hand clinical data in detail, and individualize the examination plan and treatment plan, so as to avoid the intervention provider from becoming an "unrealistic intervention provider."

William Osler, the father of modern medicine, once said, "To study the phenomenon of disease without books is to sail an uncharted sea, while to study books without patients is not to go to sea at all." Professor Zhang Xiaoqian, a famous doctor in China, also believes that the greatest feature of clinical medicine is that it cannot leave the practice and the patient. It is important to go deep into the patients, rather than simply putting effort into the books. Patients are the best teachers, and the growth of an excellent intervention provider cannot be achieved without learning from patients. When developing clinical thinking skills, we should use the knowledge we have to analyze and judge flexibly according to the actual situation of patients' conditions and should not be "book-oriented," because an intervention provider who is far from clinical practice will only be a theoretician and will never be able to improve clinical thinking and skills.

2.3.3 Scientific Thinking

The methodology of scientific research can be summarized in the following steps: data collection and organization, statistical analysis, hypothesis formulation, experimental design, experimental completion, and drawing conclusions. The diagnosis and treatment process of intervention providers should be like doing scientific research, starting from the collection of clinical data, proposing hypothetical diagnosis on the basis of induction, summary, and analysis, verifying it in further examination and treatment, and finally proposing a treatment plan. Intervention providers need to treat each case with scientific and rigorous methods, and if scientific research methods can be consciously applied to clinical thinking, the clinical thinking ability can be greatly improved. In the process of integrating the scientific research thinking mode into the clinical thinking mode, surgical intervention providers need to be familiar with all aspects of scientific research: how to collect and analyze data, how to summarize, propose, and revise the diagnosis, how to individualize the treatment plan according to specific patients, how to track and pay attention to the progress and development frontiers of the discipline, and integrate the scientific spirit, rigorous attitude, and awareness of exploration into the diagnosis and treatment process.

2.3.4 Keeping Pace with the Times

Firstly, clinical thinking needs to shift from "disease-centered" to "patient-centered." Because the object of medical treatment is specific patients, rather than abstract diseases, the traditional treatment model of seeing the disease is no longer able to adapt to the current treatment needs. In addition to physical disease, patients also need care and treatment in psychological and sociological aspects. In addition to paying attention to the treatment of the disease itself, clinical thinking must also contain psychological and social factors. Only through the organic combination of biological, psychological, social, and humanistic, a good therapeutic effect can be obtained. If the intervention provider does not consider the patient's psychological factors and social environment and only considers the treatment needs of the disease, it is difficult to obtain the patient's trust and cooperation during the treatment, and the treatment effect will be greatly reduced.

Secondly, with the rapid change of diagnosis, treatment means, and technology, the compliant treatment concept and thinking mode have been unable to adapt to the development and progress of medicine. Intervention providers need to continuously update knowledge theory and learn new skills and means in order to better improve the level of diagnosis and treatment and promote the continuous update and improvement of clinical thinking. For example, the emergence of three-dimensional reconstruction technology in the diagnosis greatly shortens the learning curve of preoperative reading of surgical intervention providers, improves the preoperative analysis ability of the condition, facilitates the early prediction of possible risks, and proposes a detailed surgical plan to avoid risks in advance. In the treatment, with the application of intraoperative fluorescence imaging technology, as well as the promotion and dissemination of minimally invasive techniques such as laparoscopy and robotics, some previous invasive surgeries requiring laparotomy have been able to be completed in a minimally invasive manner, which not only reduces the physical trauma of patients, but also reduces the psychological blow and promotes the rapid recovery of patients. In addition, the comprehensive treatment of cancer represented by targeted drugs and immunotherapy has developed rapidly and significantly, which brings dawn to the long-term survival of cancer patients after surgery and improves the quality of life. If the clinical thinking of intervention providers cannot closely follow the change and progress of medical technology and concept, it will certainly fail to meet the growing demand for precision treatment of patients.

3 Application of Evidence-Based Medicine

Traditional medicine is based on experience and relies on the experience and intuition of the intervention provider for diagnosis and treatment. However, individual experience is limited and cannot accumulate a large number of comprehensive cases in a short period of time. With only one-sided understanding of diseases and non-experimental clinical experience, it is impossible to comprehensively understand the law of disease occurrence and development, nor it can meet people's pursuit of health care in the new era, nor it can accurately guide clinical decisions.

Medicine is a science of practice. In the era of positivism, the decision of intervention providers is increasingly dependent on evidence, in which case evidence-based medicine emerges. Evidence-based medicine correctly evaluates each aspect of clinical decision-making by following high-quality clinical research evidence. Evidence-based medicine does not deny the clinical experience, clinical skills, and medical expertise of intervention providers, but only emphasizes that any clinical decision should be based on the best scientific research evidence, and its purpose is to make the clinical decision of intervention providers more perfect, accurate, and scientific. Evidence from clinical research must be combined with the specific condition of the patient, the experience of the intervention provider, and the wishes of the patient.

3.1 Concept

Evidence-based medicine is the best research basis that can be obtained cautiously, accurately, and wisely applied at present. At the same time, combining with the personal professional skills of intervention providers and many years of clinical experience, considering the value and desire of patients, the three are perfectly combined to develop the treatment measures for patients.

There are three main factors that constitute the decision-making model of evidence-based medicine: (1) Macroscopic laws and regulations, social norms, medical security system, and other factors; (2) Objective basic medical research evidence, clinical randomized controlled trials, systematic review, and the specific condition of patients; (3) Subjective clinical experience and skills of intervention providers, the cultural level, religious beliefs, and value orientation of patients and other factors. The interaction of the above factors constitutes the clinical decision-making system of evidence-based medicine.

3.2 Clinical Applications

3.2.1 To Establish the Thinking of Evidence-Based Medicine

In complex clinical decision-making, intervention providers often encounter a variety of selection problems, such as the diagnostic methods of difficult cases, indications for innovative therapies, selection and standardization of intervention means, and how to individualize and optimize treatment, which are far from enough based on personal experience alone. Many medical decisions have a double-edged sword effect, with the potential for both patient benefit and risk and harm, making it difficult to strike a balance. Therefore, it is necessary to follow the evidence-based medical model in clinical practice, based on the search for scientific evidence and evaluation of its effectiveness and practicality, propose a set of continuously improved criteria and methods that combine the individualized situation of patients and the clinical experience of physicians, in order to make the most optimal clinical decisions under the existing medical conditions.

The thinking mode of evidence-based medicine is different from the traditional thinking mode based on personal experience and book theory in the past, but advocates that the establishment of any medical decision is based on the combination of medical technology, patient needs, and best evidence. Therefore, intervention providers need to actively establish the new thinking of evidence-based medicine, consciously integrate the concept of evidence-based medicine into clinical decision-making, strengthen the awareness of matching with the Internet big data era, so that evidence-based medicine truly becomes a practical tool for intervention providers to carry out clinical decision-making, which is also the only way to closely follow the development of medical science and technology.

3.2.2 To Make Clinical Decisions Based on Evidence-Based Medical Evidence

The core idea of evidence-based medicine is to rely on evidence for decision-making, use various data obtained in clinical diagnosis and treatment, rely on statistical methods for processing, transformation, analysis, and then be utilized by researchers according to needs and applied in clinical decision-making practice. When we encounter complex cases in the medical process, have doubts in the diagnosis and treatment process, or need to evaluate the medical behavior, we need to be good at taking advantage of the development advantages of the Internet and big data, search for the best current evidence-based medical evidence, and provide the best treatment plan for patients. Excellent intervention providers should have both rich clinical experience and the ability to apply evidence-based medical evidence to guide clinical practice, both of which are indispensable.

Evidence-based medicine requires intervention providers to take evidence-based medical evidence as the guiding principle for the diagnosis and treatment of patients, especially in some controversial clinical decision-making fields, actively apply the principle of evidence-based medicine to carry out clinical trials with high evidence level, and select more reasonable treatment strategies according to the clinical benefits of patients. When facing the puzzle of selecting the treatment method, we can search the relevant clinical study literatures from Medline and Pubmed, then evaluate the literatures of different treatment methods, remove some false positive results caused by lack of repeatability or selection bias, try to select the randomized controlled study results, and systematically evaluate and statistically combine these results. And combine the results of the study that will be obtained with the intervention provider's own experience and level and the specific condition and needs of the patient, select the most appropriate treatment option for that patient. For example, it has been debated in clinical practice whether standard lymph node dissection including groups 13, 17, and 12 lymph nodes or extended lymph node dissection including groups 8, 9, 13, 17, 12, 14, and 16 lymph nodes as well as the plexus on the right side of the celiac trunk and superior mesenteric artery is performed in patients with pancreatic head cancer undergoing radical surgery. A randomized controlled study of 167 patients in 7 centers on the above issues showed that extended lymph node dissection did not bring significant survival benefit compared with standard lymph node dissection, but led to an increased incidence of postoperative complications and delayed postoperative recovery, so standard lymph node dissection may be a more reasonable treatment strategy for patients with pancreatic head cancer.

3.2.3 To Timely Grasp the Progress of Evidence-Based Medicine

Since evidence-based medicine is in continuous development and progress, through the continuous development, induction, and summary of high-level evidence research, there will be new clinical treatment options or concepts proposed and confirmed, so the conclusion of evidence-based medicine is not static, but in continuous update and development, in clinical practice, in addition to using the principles and methods of evidence-based medicine to guide clinical decision-making, timely grasp the latest progress of evidence-based medicine to promote the progress and development of medical technology and treatment concepts in this field. For example, for the application of endoscopic therapy including EMR and ESD techniques in the treatment of early gastric cancer, early retrospective study scholars with a large sample found that in some patients with early gastric cancer, endoscopic therapy can obtain the same long-term prognosis as traditional surgery. However, due to the lack of confirmation with other prospective studies compared with other surgery methods, the absolute indication of endoscopic therapy is strictly grasped in various countries, and it is not recommended as a conventional treatment. It is only limited to tumors limited to the mucosa with diameter $\leq$ 2 cm. Next, Japanese scholars conducted a large-sample prospective study on the expanded indications of ESD for early gastric cancer, and the results confirmed that ESD for early gastric cancer of intestinal type, limited to mucosa, without ulcer diameter > 2 cm or with ulcer diameter $\leq$ 3 cm was safe and effective. On the basis of evidence-based medical guidance, endoscopic treatment of early gastric cancer breaks through the bottleneck of development and further determines its role and scope of indications in the treatment of early gastric cancer. For another example, most previous retrospective studies have shown that mild hypothermia treatment can effectively reduce intracranial pressure in patients with severe head injury, but multicenter prospective randomized controlled trials designed according to the principle of evidence-based medicine believe that mild hypothermia treatment has no obvious advantage in reducing intracranial pressure, not only cannot improve the prognosis of patients but will increase the risk of systemic complications, so the study of mild hypothermia treatment in patients with severe head injury has stagnated. The latest multicenter prospective randomized controlled study stratified patients with severe head injury. The results showed that mild hypothermia treatment had a significant effect on patients with GCS 6 ~ 8, younger than 45 years old and reaching hypothermia level within 6 h, which could significantly improve the prognosis of patients. This brought new vitality to mild hypothermia treatment and pointed out a new direction for further clinical application.

How to evaluate whether a treatment is safe and effective, and how to plan out the range of indications for a certain therapy requires researchers to adopt the method of evidence-based medicine and gradually clarify it through long-term, large-sample clinical studies, which is a long process and cannot be achieved overnight. Only after a large number of clinical practice tests we can avoid unnecessary harm to patients caused by empirical blind abuse, and only by mastering the continuous updating of evidence-based medicine we can promote better development and improvement of clinical medicine.

3.2.4 To Establish Evidence-Based Medicine Decision-Making System

Evidence-based medicine needs to be based on scientific evidence based on clinical problems; therefore, the formation of evidence-based medicine decision-making system needs to go through the following five stages: (1) questions raising. Propose evidence-based clinical problems for specific patients, which can involve etiology, diagnosis, treatment, prognosis, and other aspects. (2) Evidences search.

Evidence-based clinical questions are asked for specific patients that can address etiology, diagnosis, treatment, prognosis, etc. (3) Evidence assessment. The authenticity, reliability, and availability of the research evidence are evaluated. (4) Clinical application. The results of the evidence are applied to clinical practice in conjunction with the intervention provider's clinical experience and the patient's personal needs. Of course, not all clinical questions can be found with the highest level of evidence, but sources of evidence with high levels of rank and recommendation should be used whenever possible. (5) System evaluation. Track and analyze the application effect of clinical decision-making, verify the reliability, practicability, and validity of evidence through clinical practice, and make a rational evaluation.

In the process of establishing evidence-based medicine decision-making system, it is also necessary to consider various factors affecting the composition of decision-making, such as the reliability of evidence sources, the scientificity of research methods, the compliance of patients and the support of external environment. Under the condition of eliminating the influence of various abnormal factors, in order to obtain the most reliable evidence and make an objective and accurate evaluation, a clinical guidance system based on scientific evidence can be established to form a diagnosis and treatment specification for some specific diseases and specific treatment methods, and new scientific evidence can be formed to guide clinical practice.

3.2.5 Individualized Practice of Evidence-Based Medicine

Individualized treatment is the process by which intervention providers take appropriate medical measures for patients according to their specific conditions, combining with scientific evidence, clinical experience, or pathophysiological reasoning. In clinical practice, intervention providers face the following problems every day: the symptoms and signs of patients are not consistent with those described in textbooks, the disease stage of patients is not completely consistent with the staging of guidelines, and the rules on textbooks and guidelines are difficult to be applied for the diagnostic basis and treatment methods.

The evidence and conclusions provided by evidence-based medicine are common principles and can guide clinical decision-making, but this is not contradictory to individualized treatment, and even more effective than traditional medical decision-making methods to carry out individualized treatment. The concept of evidence-based medicine itself emphasizes the individualization of science and requires the consideration of many factors such as clinical research evidence, the experience of intervention providers, and the wishes of patients. Correct weighting of evidence, experience, and other factors in the treatment of different patients is key to selecting individualized treatment options.

At present, evidence-based medicine is still in the primary stage of development, there are still a large number of clinical problems without scientific answers in medical practice, and a considerable number of diagnosis and treatment methods lack reliable research evidence. When there is no reference research evidence for the special condition of patients, non-randomized controlled studies, expert consensus, experience, and pathophysiological mechanism reasoning can be used as the reference basis for decision-making, and the feasibility and cost-effectiveness ratio of intervention measures can be comprehensively assessed in combination with factors such as side effects, costs, and patient wishes of treatment, and evidence can be achieved as much as possible. With the development of medicine, high-quality clinical research evidence continues to increase, and intervention providers can guide the formulation of individualized clinical decisions for patients through the continuous improvement and revision of the evidence-based medicine system.

3.3 Limitations of Evidence-Based Medicine

Evidence-based medicine emphasizes that medical decisions must be based on clinical research results while considering the subjective needs of patients, and its purpose is to reduce the interference of intervention provider subjective factors on disease treatment through objective evidence. Therefore, evidence-based medicine approaches focus on studying the relationship between interventions and disease risk, and interventions also replace intervention providers as a major factor interacting with disease risk and affecting prognosis.

In the intervention for disease risk, empirical medicine relies too much on intervention providers, while evidence-based medicine overcorrects empirical medicine and overemphasizes the choice of intervention means while ignoring the intervention providers' mastery of intervention means and the important impact on the prognosis of patients. Although Professor David Sackett, the founder of evidence-based medicine, added that evidence-based medicine should "combine the personal professional skills and years of clinical experience of intervention providers" in the concept of the latest edition of evidence-based medicine in 2000, the limitation of its research method determines that evidence-based medicine is difficult to objectively include intervention provider factors in the research category. For example, in the treatment of small liver cancer, evidence-based medical evidence recommends surgery as the first choice of treatment, but evidence-based medical evidence only considers that surgery, an intervention, can achieve the best therapeutic effect, but does not consider whether the intervention provider has the ability and experience to perform liver surgery. If the intervention provider is not good at surgical treatment, it is obviously not a wise choice to select the intervention according to evidence-based medical evidence.

3.4 Significance

Evidence-based medicine is of great significance in the formulation of clinical decisions and improving the prognosis of patients. The purpose of evidence-based medicine is to solve clinical problems. By combining and comprehensively analyzing the collection of objective medical research evidence, the accumulation of clinical work experience and skills, and the medical needs of different patients, the accuracy of diagnosis and the rationality of treatment can be effectively improved. In the implementation process of prognosis control surgery, we fully attach importance to the concept of evidence-based medicine, emphasize the effective use of evidence-based medicine principles and methods, select effective and reasonable intervention means, and finally achieve the optimal prognosis of patients.

3.4.1 To Facilitate the Scientificity of Clinical Decision-Making

The application of evidence-based medicine in clinical medicine is mainly to solve various practical problems encountered in clinical medicine. Evidence-based medicine can provide a reliable basis for the early diagnosis of some diseases, especially those that seriously endanger people's health or have a poor prognosis, which can help intervention providers to provide patients with the most effective, reliable, and practical evidence of treatment after practical testing. From expert opinions at low evidence level to randomized controlled studies, systematic reviews, and meta-analyses at high evidence level, evidence-based medicine standardizes medical behavior patterns and promotes the scientificity of medical decision-making by learning from the evidence in previous clinical practice.

3.4.2 To Promote the Transformation of Medical Education Model

Practice evidence-based medicine can promote medical education from the traditional teaching model based on lecture to the evidence-based medicine model based on active search for evidence, on the one hand, it helps to cultivate the positive exploration spirit and active thinking ability of intervention providers, on the other hand, it helps to integrate the use of longitudinal drilling ability, horizontal thinking ability, the use of knowledge to solve problems, and doctor–patient communication ability. When facing a specific patient, under the training model of evidence-based medicine, intervention providers can better carry out clinical thinking, make diagnosis and treatment decisions, and can more reasonably answer various questions of patients and their families.

3.4.3 To Promote the Development of Medical Scientific Research

Evidence-based medicine can continuously find medical evidence according to specific clinical problems, so that intervention providers can comprehensively and systematically understand the current research status in a field and put it into clinical practice and can also find some unsolved clinical problems as a new research direction to provide guidance for clinical practice. Since evidence-based medicine can continuously strictly evaluate the obtained research evidence in order to apply more scientific research methods to improve the defects in the design, implementation, and discussion of previous studies, so as to promote the standardization of clinical research and the improvement of research quality.

4 Application of MDT Mode

"If a tumor patient goes to internal medicine department first, then he will undergo internal chemotherapy. If he goes to surgery first, he will perform surgery, and if he goes to radiotherapy first, he will perform radiotherapy." This example accurately and graphically illustrates the fragmented treatment status between various disciplines in the hospital, as well as the necessity of carrying out MDT (Multiple Disciplinary Team).

MDT originated in the 1940s. With the progress of medical technology and the accumulation of medical research evidence, not only the diagnosis and treatment equipment is continuously developed and used, but also the treatment strategy, concept, and model are continuously updated. The individualized treatment from general and empirical treatment methods to different diagnosis and treatment methods according to the individual characteristics of patients is excessive. In the 1990s, the UK established by legislation a model that MDT must follow for the diagnosis and treatment of malignancies. In Europe and the USA, MDT has become an important part of the hospital health care system and a normalized treatment model. The National Cancer Comprehensive Network in the USA and the National Health Care Program in the UK have included MDT in the clinical practice guidelines for a variety of diseases.

4.1 Concept and Feature

4.1.1 Definition

MDT is a clinical treatment model in which two or more related disciplines and relatively fixed expert groups make scientific, rational, and standardized treatment decisions for a certain disease or patient through regular, timed, scheduled, and site-specific multidisciplinary seminars, bringing together the latest developments in each discipline, taking into account the patient's disease stage, treatment needs, family economic conditions, physical condition, psychological ability, etc., weighing the pros and cons and then supervising the implementation of the treatment plan and regularly evaluating the efficacy and adjusting the plan to ensure maximum benefit for the patient. MDT members usually include multidisciplinary experts in surgery, internal medicine, radiotherapy, intervention, ultrasound, imaging, and pathology. Professionals in basic research, nursing, psychology and nutrition, social workers, and patient families can be important components of MDT.

MDT is a novel diagnosis and treatment model that is transformed from traditional empirical medicine to modern cooperative group decision-making on the basis of evidence-based medicine. MDT is based on the principle of patient-centered holistic treatment, with doctors from various specialties as the basis, and a patient-centered treatment model to discuss diseases, rather than the traditional disease-centered consultation. The MDT treatment model aims to maximize the benefits of treatment for patients. The MDT expert group implements individualized treatment in a scientific, rational, standardized, and planned manner in full accordance with evidence-based medical evidence, tailoring treatment to each patient rather than a one-size-fits-all approach, avoiding the need for each specialist to implement interventions only from the perspective of his or her own specialty.

4.1.2 Feature

MDT is different from the traditional consultation model, and its characteristics are mainly manifested in the following three aspects:

1. MDT is a model system with a relatively strict and standardized system and organization, time, people and place, rather than the traditional random and loose consultation model;
2. MDT selects experts from relevant specialties to participate according to the specific condition of the patient, and after multidisciplinary discussion, reaches a consensus on diagnosis and treatment with the patient, while the traditional consultation model selects experts from the patient's requirements;
3. MDT model is a diagnosis and treatment under multidisciplinary collaboration, which not only contains the diagnosis in the traditional consultation model, but also includes the selection and implementation of the diagnosis and treatment plan. During the treatment and rehabilitation process, the team of experts will regularly evaluate the effectiveness of the treatment and constantly adjust the treatment plan to make it more relevant to the patient's situation and make it easier to implement.

4.2 Necessity and Significance

4.2.1 Necessity

The Inevitable Results of the Development of Medical Science and Technology

With the development of medicine, the more and more refined professional division system makes the study of diseases more and more in-depth in the longitudinal development, has a more thorough understanding of the nature of diseases, and makes the diagnosis and treatment of diseases more specialized. However, on the other hand, the traditional single and longitudinal development model has many limitations and is easy to fall into a fragmented circle. In the face of complex and atypical clinical cases, a single discipline often cannot cope with it alone, and a single treatment method brings better diagnosis and treatment effect to patients.

At present, circulating tumor cells, liquid biopsy, genetic testing, PET-CT, and other examination methods emerge in endlessly, and the treatment methods represented by targeted drugs, biological immunotherapy, conformal radiotherapy, interventional therapy, and robotic surgery have made the diagnosis and treatment techniques of diseases change rapidly. Therefore, it is necessary to break the professional barriers between disciplines, organically combine the development frontiers of various related disciplines with the specific circumstances of patients' diseases under the guidance of evidence-based medicine principles, and develop an individualized treatment plan in line with the interests of patients through the exchange and cooperation between multiple disciplines.

Necessary Requirements for the Transformation of Medical Concept

Modern medical model has changed from biomedical model to bio-psycho-social medical model, and traditional disease-centered traditional thinking model has also changed to patient-centered humanistic medicine. Under the guidance of the prognosis control surgical concept with the goal of optimal prognosis of patients, in addition to paying attention to the treatment of the disease itself, the surgical diagnosis and treatment process also needs to include psychological and social factors to achieve an organic combination of biological, psychological, social, and humanistic in order to obtain a good therapeutic effect.

Especially in terms of cancer treatment, the treatment goal has prolonged the tumor-bearing survival time from simply pursuing the tumor-free survival time and overall survival time to maintaining the quality of life, and this disruptive change in the treatment concept requires corresponding changes in the diagnosis and treatment model. The MDT model conforms to the requirements of the development of the current era, integrates the latest achievements in the development of various disciplines, moves from traditional single closed treatment to rational and reasonable multidisciplinary cooperation, and changes from isolated and one-sided personal judgment to efficient and comprehensive collective wisdom.

Inevitable Trend of Integration and Optimization of Medical Resources

In the current informatization era, core competitiveness no longer depends on the degree and speed of personal knowledge and skills accumulation, but on the ability and level of resource integration. Intervention providers should have the awareness of effectively integrating multidisciplinary diagnosis and treatment means. However, the integration of medical resources is not to arbitrarily superpose and apply multiple diagnosis and treatment means, but to combine and give play to the advantages of various disciplines from person to person according to the physiological status, disease characteristics, development stage, and other specific circumstances of different patients.

MDT model can break the previously limited system of division by treatment means, determine the specific and appropriate treatment objectives by integrating the treatment ability of doctors and the treatment needs of patients; integrate the advanced diagnosis and treatment means in various professional fields into a feasible diagnosis and treatment plan through the cross cooperation of various disciplines, promote the mutual integration of specialization and integration, and maximize the interests of patients; ensure that various diagnosis and treatment means are carried out simultaneously or sequentially and orderly through regular supervision, make the medical process more accurate, efficient, and humanized, and promote the optimal allocation and use of medical resources.

4.2.2 Significance

MDT model truly reflects the advantages of multidisciplinary cooperation and standardized treatment, effectively avoids the limitations caused by the tubular thinking of professional physicians, and each professional discipline no longer fights alone.

By integrating the academic advantages of multidisciplinary, the accuracy and early diagnosis rate of diagnosis are improved to the greatest extent, a reasonable and standardized treatment plan is developed, and the optimal individualized diagnosis and treatment plan is provided for patients. MDT model achieves a seamless multi-disciplinary link related to the disease, eliminates the differences in the understanding of guidelines and norms among specialties, and realizes individualized and precise diagnosis and treatment on the basis of standardization, thus ensuring the maximization of patient benefits and promoting the optimal allocation of medical resources.

MDT model builds a learning and exchange platform combining relevant disciplines, theory and practice frontiers, and clinical and medical technology, which can not only broaden the vision of specialist physicians, deepen their understanding of the latest progress of relevant specialties, form clinical thinking with a holistic view and a general view, promote the interdisciplinary development, improve the medical level of various specialties, subspecialties, and the overall medical level, provide more comprehensive and profound diagnosis and treatment experience, and directly promote the overall improvement of medical level.

4.3 Clinical Applications

4.3.1 Stratified Management Is Performed for Patients

MDT requires focused multidisciplinary discussion of difficult cases that most require MDT within a limited period of time, so strict and detailed inclusion criteria need to be developed, and patients need to be distinguished and classified at the time of initial diagnosis to exert the maximum effect of MDT and also allow patients to obtain the greatest benefit.

4.3.2 Ensure Regular MDT Consultations

When MDT is carried out, it is necessary to have a specially assigned person responsible for convening and implementing it, so as to ensure that senior physicians in various disciplines can attend the consultation and participate in the discussion on time. In MDT consultation and discussion, the will of patients and their families should be fully considered, evidence-based medical evidence from various disciplines and diagnosis and treatment progress should be organically combined, and basic contents such as clinical decision-making, clarifying disease diagnosis, determining treatment plan, evaluating the implementation effect, and timely revising should be formulated.

4.3.3 Good Management and Quality Control Are Conducted for MDT Cases

MDT should be standardized and normalized in terms of procedure and content. All patients undergoing MDT need to have detailed and traceable case data. The case management of MDT covers the process of patient evaluation, diagnosis, treatment, and connection between various treatments. In the process of initial diagnosis, admitting doctors should improve the collection and filing of clinical case data to achieve accuracy. During the MDT consultation discussion, the treating physician should record in detail each differential diagnosis, diagnostic basis, and treatment plan. In the MDT treatment process, the treating physician shall record in detail and timely feedback the completion of treatment plan, adverse reactions, and treatment measures of the patient in charge, organize the institution to supervise and monitor the implementation of diagnosis and treatment plan, and regularly improve and optimize the MDT management system and protocol process. After the end of MDT, a follow-up plan should be developed to pay attention to the efficacy, prognosis, and psychological changes of patients and timely feedback the treatment effect of patients to MDT organization in the form of email, SMS, and telephone, so as to evaluate and summarize the experience and lessons of treatment.

4.3.4 Adhere to the Patient-Centered Principle

It should fully consider the views, wishes, and needs of patients and their families during the implementation of MDT, respect the right to know and the right to choose and decide the treatment plan of patients and their families, develop the final diagnosis and treatment plan through communication with patients and their families, and strictly implement it. All feasible treatment options should be considered during the discussion, and some active treatment methods should not be abandoned due to the limitation of technical conditions of the hospital or the age and economic factors of the patient. For cases with incomplete information or incomplete examination results that cannot develop a clear protocol, another time may be selected for another MDT discussion.

4.4 Analysis of MDT Cases

The patient was male and 48 years old. He was admitted due to melena for 1 month and the examination revealed liver mass and sigmoid colon mass for 5 days. History of present illness: The patient had melena accompanied by feeling of incomplete evacuation without obvious inducement 1 month ago, and colonoscopy performed in a local hospital 5 days ago showed sigmoid colon mass, and pathology revealed moderately differentiated adenocarcinoma. Contrast-enhanced CT examination of the abdomen revealed multiple liver masses, considering liver metastases. Since the onset of the disease, the patient had loss of appetite, fatigue, weight loss of about 4 kg in the past 1 month, no abdominal pain or distension, no chills or high fever, no nausea or vomiting, normal urination, and normal sleep. Physical examination: The abdomen was flat, no gastrointestinal type or peristaltic waves were observed, no tenderness or rebound tenderness was observed in the whole abdomen, no palpable abdomen, liver and spleen were not palpable under the ribs, bowel sounds were normal, and no mass was palpable on digital examination. Auxiliary examination: Colonoscopy showed a large ulcerated bulge in the sigmoid colon 30 cm from the anus, invading the intestinal lumen for 3/5 weeks, pathologically moderately differentiated adenocarcinoma, and K-ras gene detection was wild-type. Contrast-enhanced CT of the abdomen showed multiple low-density tumors in the liver (maximum about 8 cm × 8 cm × 5 cm), annular enhancement in the arterial phase of the lesion in the liver parenchyma, thickening of the intestinal wall of the sigmoid colon, clear retroperitoneal structure, and no enlarged lymph nodes. Lung CT showed no significant abnormality. Routine blood tests and biochemical tests showed no significant abnormalities. CEA 90.5 ng/mL, CA19-9 930.3 U/mL, KPS score: 90, ECOG score: 1.

The first MDT discussion: The opinions of the Department of General Surgery and the Department of Hepatobiliary Surgery were as follows: Combined with the current examination results, the patient was diagnosed with sigmoid colon cancer with multiple liver metastases. Referring to the seventh edition of the AJCC staging criteria, the patient's tumor stage was T3N0M1a. In this case, as assessed by the Department of Hepatobiliary Surgery, it was considered that multiple liver metastases were distributed in both the left and right lobes, and the largest metastasis invaded the middle hepatic vein, which was potentially resectable, but the possibility of positive resection margin was high. After general surgery evaluation, the primary tumor of the sigmoid colon was considered clear and no significant metastatic lymph nodes were seen on imaging, and minimally invasive laparoscopic surgery was feasible. After medical oncology evaluation, it was considered that such patients should be treated systemically first according to NCCN guidelines, and sigmoid resection should be considered only when there is a significant risk of intestinal obstruction or hematochezia. The available regimens were FOLFIRI/FOLFOX/CapeOX ± bevacizumab or FOLFIRI ± cetuximab or FOLFIRIOX. Given that the K-ras was wild-type, the highest recommended regimen was FOLFIRI + cetuximab. If the lesion was expected to convert to resectability, an assessment of whether it could be operated was performed every 2 months. After multidisciplinary consultation and comprehensive discussion with the patient's family, it was decided to perform preoperative neoadjuvant therapy for the patient.

After 6 weeks of FOLFIRI plus cetuximab treatment, the patient developed mild skin toxicity (local papulopustular reaction), which improved with local treatment. CEA 23.8 ng/mL, CA19-9 115.6 U/mL. Reexamination of enhanced CT of the liver showed that the largest metastasis had been significantly reduced, located in the right liver, about 1 cm away from the middle hepatic vein, and the left liver metastasis had disappeared. Reexamination of enteroscopy showed that the lesion was reduced and the ulcer surface became shallower. After neoadjuvant therapy, the tumor markers decreased significantly, and the tumor was significantly relieved by imaging and endoscopic observation, suggesting that the patient was sensitive to this treatment regimen.

The second MDT discussion: The expert group discussed together and decided to perform one-stage surgical treatment. The Department of General Surgery combined with the Department of Hepatobiliary Surgery performed laparoscopic radical resection of sigmoid colon cancer combined with right hemihepatectomy for the patient. Intraoperative ultrasound exploration of the liver was applied and no obvious metastases were seen in the left half of the liver. Multiple metastases were located in the right half of the liver and laparoscopic right hepatectomy was performed in the hepatobiliary surgery with adequate hemostasis of the wound and the resected specimen was placed in a sterile protective sleeve and placed under the liver for removal. Laparoscopic radical resection of sigmoid colon cancer was performed by the Department of General Surgery. Postoperative pathology revealed ulcerated moderately differentiated adenocarcinoma (6 cm × 3 cm), invading the subserosa, upper and lower resection margins (−), mesenteric lymph nodes 0/15 (−), hemangioma emboli (−), nerve invasion (+), lymphangioma emboli (+), multiple metastatic adenocarcinomas in the right liver tissue, and hemangioma emboli (−). The patient was able to get out of bed on the second day after surgery, had anal exhaust on the third day after surgery, and was discharged on the seventh day after surgery. At 4 weeks after operation, CEA: 10.5 ng/mL, CA199:18.6 U/mL, abdominopelvic enhanced CT showed no significant abnormality. The patient was advised to continue chemotherapy combined with targeted therapy after surgery, but after communicating with the patient and his family, the patient and his family refused further treatment.

At 12 weeks after surgery, the patient was found to have a mass in the left medial lobe of the liver by reexamination of abdominal contrast-enhanced CT, considering new metastases, measuring about 2 cm × 1 cm. The right adrenal tumor measured about 2.5 cm × 3.5 cm, considering the possibility of new metastases. PET-CT examination showed a round mass in the left medial lobe of the liver, measuring about 2.3 cm × 1.5 cm, showing significant abnormal radioactive concentration, SUVmax 8.2, and a round mass shadow in the right adrenal region, measuring 3.1 cm × 3.8 cm, showing significant abnormal radioactive concentration, SUVmax 7.6. CEA 38.8 ng/mL, CA19-9 135.5 U/mL. After evaluation by the imaging department, it was considered that postoperative liver and adrenal recurrence was considered in combination with the patient's imaging data and tumor markers.

The third MDT discussion: Opinion of the Department of Hepatobiliary Surgery: the patient was considered to have a new metastasis, the tumor was single and located in the left medial lobe. Second surgery was more invasive, and the patient was recommended to undergo radiofrequency ablation. Urological opinion: The new tumor was located in the right adrenal gland, and there was no obvious adhesion or invasion between the tumor and the surrounding organs. Advice of medical oncology: The patient should continue the previous treatment plan to 6 courses after surgery. The current reexamination results suggest recurrence of liver and adrenal gland. Given that the patient's colon tumor K-ras was wild-type and that the FOLFIRI plus cetuximab regimen was effective preoperatively, the FOLFIRI plus cetuximab regimen could be continued. Hepatobiliary surgery combined with urology percutaneous transhepatic left medial lobe radiofrequency ablation combined with retroperitoneoscopic right adrenalectomy. During the operation, a single tumor of about 3.5 cm × 4.1 cm in size was observed in the right adrenal gland, without obvious adhesion to the surrounding, or atrophy of the surrounding adrenal glands. After the tumor was fully freed, the right adrenal gland was completely removed together with the tumor. Postoperative pathology revealed metastatic adenocarcinoma of the left liver and metastatic adenocarcinoma of the right adrenal gland, which was consistent with colorectal cancer metastasis in combination with clinical history and morphology. The patient recovered well after surgery and was discharged uneventfully 4 days after surgery. Tumor markers decreased rapidly on reexamination 1 week after surgery. Two weeks after surgery, the patient began to receive standardized FOLFIRI + cetuximab treatment for 6 courses, and tumor markers, abdominopelvic enhanced CT and lung CT examinations were regularly monitored. No recurrence or metastasis was been observed so far.

With the progress of medical technology, radical hepatectomy centered on liver metastasis of colon cancer was currently a clinically recognized treatment plan. Surgery should strive to achieve no residual cancer cells at the resection margin, and radical resection should be performed as far as possible, which can significantly improve the 5-year survival rate after surgery. Colon cancer with adrenal metastasis usually lacks specific clinical symptoms, and surgical resection is the treatment of choice for adrenal metastasis of colon cancer and radical resection should be performed as early as possible. In this case, the diagnosis and treatment process was tortuous, and the patient had multiple liver metastases that were difficult to remove at the time of treatment. After MDT consultation and discussion, according to the patient's general condition, examination results, surgical evaluation and the treatment wishes of the patient and his family, the sensitive chemotherapy combined with translational therapy of targeted drugs was first selected according to the tumor gene mutation, which successfully reduced the liver metastases and primary colon tumors and obtained the chance of radical surgery. Since the patient and his family did not continue further treatment after surgery, liver and adrenal metastases recurred after surgery. After MDT discussion again and comprehensive injury-benefit ratio, two minimally invasive treatment methods, radiofrequency ablation of liver tumors and retroperitoneoscopic right adrenalectomy, were selected, which not only achieved the effect of radical treatment on the one hand, but also improved the patient's tolerance to further treatment on the other hand. After standard systemic chemotherapy combined with targeted therapy, there has been no recurrence so far. The patient with liver metastasis of colon cancer and postoperative multiple organ metastasis achieved good quality of life and survival benefit through a series of means including translational therapy, combined colon cancer and liver surgery, radiofrequency ablation of recurrent liver tumors, retroperitoneoscopic resection of adrenal metastases, and postoperative chemotherapy combined with targeted therapy, fully reflecting the advantages of multidisciplinary cooperation model in individualized treatment and reflecting the crystallization of collective wisdom.

Suggested Reading

Chen MJ, Zhang JD, Wen DX, Liang C, Sun XF. Current status and countermeasures of multidisciplinary diagnosis and treatment model of cancer based on the perspective of doctors. Chin Hosp. 2016;20(8):39–43.

Evidence-Based Medicine Working Group. Evidence-based medicine. A new approach to teaching the practice of medicine. JAMA. 1992;268(17):2420–5.

Feng BX. Concepts, techniques, and arts of surgical decision making. Med Philos. 2007.

Gao YX. The impact of evidence-based medicine on clinical decision-making. Med Information. 2007;2:110–4.

Gu J. Decision making of surgeons. Chin J Pract Surg. 2008;28(7):527–8.

Guyatt G. Evidence-based decision-making is individualized clinical decision-making. Chin J Evid Based Med. 2007;7(2):93–9.

He QY. How to scientifically formulate clinical decision-making - evidence-based medicine, guideline consensus, precision medicine, integrated medicine and clinical decision-making. Med Philos. 2016;37(6B):1–4.

Hua W. Evidence-based medicine and practice. Chin J Evid Based Cardiovasc Med. 2010;2(4):252–3.

Hua CJ, Hao H. Current status and prospect of multidisciplinary consultation for oncology. Med Recapitulate. 2015;21(3):431–5.

Huang ZQ. About surgical decision-making. J Chin PLA Postgrad Med School. 2012;33(3):201–10.

Latifi R. Surgical decision making- beyond the evidence based surgery. Cham: Springer; 2016.

Liu YX. The core of surgical clinical decision-making is proficiency in selection. Med Philos. 2006a;27(5):1–3.

Liu DW. Clinical thinking in surgical critical care assessment. Chin J Surg. 2006b;44(17):1166.

Liu M. Clinical individualization should be based on evidence-based decision-making as much as possible. Chin J Evid Based Med. 2007;7(2):83–4.

Liu SL, Fan J, Tang WH, Wang EH, Sun MY. Clinical thinking of surgical intervention providers. Med Philos. 1999;20(2):44–6.

Min JH, Kang TW, Cha DI, Song KD, Lee MW, Rhim H, Sinn DH, Kim JM, Sohn I. Radiofrequency ablation versus surgical resection for multiple HCCs meeting the Milan criteria: propensity score analyses of 10-year therapeutic outcomes. Clin Radiol. 2018;73(7):676.e15–24.

Specialized Committee of Gastrointestinal Oncology, Chinese Research Hospital Association, Specialized Committee of Multidisciplinary Comprehensive Therapy, Chinese College of Surgeons. Expert consensus on the diagnosis and treatment model of Multidisciplinary Treatment Collaborative Group for Digestive Tract Tumors. Chin J Pract Surg. 2017;37(1):30–1.

Wang YQ. Paying attention to cultivating good surgical clinical thinking style. Chin J Pract Surg. 2006;26(1):2–4.

Xia HS. Clinical thinking of surgical intervention providers. Mod Clin Gen Surg. 1996;1(2):65–7.

Xu XL, Liu XD, Liang M, Luo BM. Radiofrequency ablation versus hepatic resection for small hepatocellular carcinoma: systematic review of randomized controlled trials with meta-analysis and trial sequential analysis. Radiology. 2018;287(2):461–72.

Yamao T, Imai K, Yamashita YI, Kaida T, Nakagawa S, Mima K, Hashimoto D, Chikamoto A, Ishiko T, Baba H. Surgical treatment strategy for hepatocellular carcinoma in patients with impaired liver function: hepatic resection or radiofrequency ablation? HPB (Oxford). 2018;20(3):244–50.

Yan XY, Dong YC, Yao C. Evidence-based medicine research in the era of big data. Chin J Evid Based Med. 2017;17(3):249–54.

Yang Z, Qiu FZ. Surgical clinical decision-making. Chin J Pract Surg. 2007;27(1):19–22.

Zeng XJ. Training of young surgeons. J Pract Surg. 1984;4(1):55–6.

Zhang DQ. Clinical decision-making: an important field of medical philosophy research. Med Philos. 2004;25(12):17–21.

Zhang JX. Clinical decision and information redundancy. Zhonghua Yi Xue Za Zhi. 2005;85(32):2236–7.

Zhang TP, Cao Z, Zhao YP. Value of multidisciplinary diagnosis and treatment model in comprehensive diagnosis and treatment decision of pancreatic cancer. Chin J Bases Clin Gen Surg. 2017;24(6):665–8.

Zhao JP, Duan WY, Cheng QY, Liang XJ. Establishment and application of evidence-based medicine decision-making model. Hosp Admin J Chin People's Liber Army. 2003;10(4):345–6.

Zhao Y, Liu YF, Hu HT, Zou Y, Piao HZ, Zhang Y, Luo YH, Bai H. The experience of promoting the multidisciplinary integrated diagnosis and treatment model in oncology specialty hospitals. China Cancer. 2014;23(12):973–8.

Optimization of Interventions

4

Rong Liu and Qu Liu

Abstract

With the development of medical technology and information technology, surgical interventions are emerging. This chapter describes how to optimize interventions in four areas: damage control, theoretical innovation, path module, and cost-effectiveness. In the section on damage control, the three main characteristics of damage control, namely rapid, minimally invasive, and precise, are described, as well as the three main categories of pathway damage control, target damage control, and additional damage control. In the section on theoretical innovation, the three major characteristic features of practical, open, and practical theoretical innovation are described, as well as the three major classifications of developmental theoretical innovation, revisional theoretical innovation, and autonomous theoretical innovation. Path mode optimization has three advantages: procedural, standardized, and efficient, and four categories: pathing of clinical diagnosis and treatment, standardization of auxiliary operation, patterning of intervention means, and modularization of complex operations. Path module optimization also needs to be summarized from clinical practice, experience summary, and practical application. Cost-benefit optimization includes cost-effective analysis, cost-utility analysis, and cost-benefit analysis. Finally, the development of artificial intelligence is reviewed.

R. Liu (✉) · Q. Liu
Faculty of Hepato-pancreato-biliary Surgery, Chinese PLA General Hospital, Beijing, China
e-mail: liurong301@126.com

R. Liu (ed.), *Clinical Decision Making for Improving Prognosis*,
https://doi.org/10.1007/978-981-19-2952-6_4

1 Damage Control Optimization

With the gradual deepening of the understanding of diseases and the continuous development of medical science and technology, the means of intervention are becoming richer and richer, and the fundamental core of its development lies in how to control losses within the minimum range. Disease risk management as a means of achieving prognosis control surgery includes both disease risk and intervention risk. How to keep both disease risk and intervention risk to a minimum in risk management, with minimal trauma in exchange for the fastest recovery for the patient, is the first consideration for the intervention provider.

1.1 Concept

Damage control was first proposed on the basis of treatment experience in patients with severe multiple trauma. The concept of damage control believes that the second hit brought about by complex surgery in patients with severe trauma will aggravate the body's ischemia and hypoxia resulting in multiple organ failure. Simple and effective controlled surgery should be performed first to quickly solve life-threatening problems such as bleeding and infection, followed by resuscitation, timely adjustment of the body's internal environment, hemodynamics, acid-base balance, coagulation dysfunction and other pathophysiological changes, and then the implementation of definitive surgery.

The traditional surgical concept usually emphasizes a one-time operation to solve all the problems of patients, for example, the treatment of liver metastases from colon cancer recommends a one-stage completion of radical resection of colon cancer combined with resection of liver metastases. However, when the patient's condition is critical, the body tolerance is poor or the surgical trauma is large, the damage caused by the surgery itself is also very serious, often bringing a second blow other than the disease to the patient. The postoperative patients are often difficult to recover due to shock, DIC, ARDS, and MODS, with a high mortality rate.

Traditional loss control is a surgical strategy for staged repair in patients with severe trauma, aiming to avoid irreversible physiological depletion due to the mutual promotion of the fatal triad (hypothermia, coagulopathy, metabolic acidosis). The damage control optimization of the intervention we propose further emphasizes that rapid control of losses, protection of tissue function, and improvement of the patient's quality of life during the diagnosis and treatment of patients are the ultimate purposes of clinical intervention. The core idea of damage control surgery lies in rapidly controlling the complex and critical primary disease of patients while avoiding the second blow and damage caused by excessive treatment operation and too long operation time and avoiding the situation that "the operation is completed and the person dies." Intervention providers need to repeatedly weigh the relationship between treatment and benefit, control risks within a controllable range, achieve optimal target damage with minimal path damage, and achieve optimal clinical benefit with minimal treatment costs.

1.2 Development History

Damage control was first used in severe trauma, especially in the treatment of war damages. In 1983, Stone et al. retrospectively reviewed the treatment experience of 31 patients with severe trauma complicated with coagulopathy and first proposed the damage control theory, arguing that in the early stage of severe trauma, in order to maintain the stability of the patient's internal environment, reduce the second blow caused by surgery, taking simple and quick measures to temporarily control the damage, and then performing staged surgery according to the actual situation of the patient after the patient's condition improves can save the critically ill patients who were originally considered unsalvageable and significantly reduce the mortality rate. In 1993, Rotondo et al. reported that the status of loss control was further determined, and the principle of three stages of loss control was gradually established: rapid control of the injury condition, continuous active resuscitation, and definitive surgery. In 2004, Finlay et al. proposed the concept of damage control laparotomy, and in 2005, Freeman et al. applied the concept of damage control surgery to the management of acute mesenteric ischemia. In recent years, the concept of damage control has been widely used in the treatment of daily trauma such as orthopedics, thoracic surgery, urology, and obstetrics and gynecology. The concept of damage control should also be widely recognized and applied in nontraumatic diseases. In 2006, Academician Li Jieshou proposed the application of the concept of damage control in the treatment of noninvasive patients, which requires the control of the damage carried by the surgery itself in addition to the control of the damage caused by the lesion.

1.3 Characteristics

1.3.1 Rapidity

The patient's condition is constantly changing, and the risks associated with it are also rapidly changing. How to grasp the best timing of treatment in limited space-time and how to optimize the risk control means to achieve damage control to the treatment means and their diseases themselves requires rapidity. The rapidity here refers not only to the rapidity of the timing of the reaction but also to the rapidity of the treatment process. Minimally invasive surgery is certainly less invasive to the patients. However, if a laparoscopic surgery takes more than 7 or 8 h, the trauma caused by that long general anesthesia and ultra-long surgical blow is much more than the trauma caused by the open incision. Even if the surgery is minimally invasive on the surface, the damage caused to the patients is actually invasive. Therefore, achieving the rapidity of interventions on the basis of long-term clinical experience accumulation and exercise is the first need for risk control.

1.3.2 Minimal Invasion

The key point of damage control emphasis lies in the control of secondary trauma caused by treatment means. Therefore, how to use minimally invasive means to achieve the control of lesions is the theme of damage control optimization. Minimal invasion here mainly refers to reducing the damage caused by the implementation of intervention paths, that is, path damage control. Taking the treatment of 3 cm liver cancer in the left lateral lobe of the liver as an example, if the left lateral lobe of the liver is removed by laparotomy, although the goal can be achieved, the trauma of the incision is huge, even exceeding the trauma endured by the liver. If the laparoscopic method can be used to complete, the minimally invasive path can be realized and the trauma caused to the patients by the large incision can be reduced.

1.3.3 Precision

On the basis of rapid and minimally invasive implementation of clinical intervention, the accuracy of disease treatment should also be emphasized to reduce the damage to the normal physiological environment and tissue function. Precision includes both the control of target damage and the control of additional damage. Target damage control refers to reduce the damage of removing the lesion to the target organs. For example, with the continuous deepening of the understanding of the anatomy of the liver, as well as the gradual application of new techniques such as three-dimensional reconstruction and fluorescence imaging, the resection of liver tumors has changed from the concept of pursuing complete resection to preserving the normal functional structural units as far as possible, protecting the liver function as far as possible while completely removing the tumor, which is conducive to the rapid recovery of patients. Additional damage control refers to reducing the additional trauma caused by intervention means, for example, the blood flow blocking of the first porta hepatis during hepatectomy will aggravate the ischemia-reperfusion damage of the remaining liver. If the blood flow into the liver lobe and segment to be removed can be accurately blocked, it will effectively reduce the damage of the remaining liver function and promote the recovery of patients.

1.4 Classification

The core content of damage control is to minimize the damage caused by surgery and various treatment methods themselves, achieve the best therapeutic effect with the least trauma, so as to accelerate the rehabilitation of patients and improve the long-term quality of life. From the perspective of medical intervention, damage control can be divided into three aspects: path damage control, target damage control, and additional damage control.

1.4.1 Path Damage Control

Path damage mainly refers to the damage caused to the body to reach the designated treatment or operation area. Such damage is not caused in the process of treatment or intervention, and often occurs before and after treatment or intervention. From the surgical point of view, the path damage control and minimal invasion concept are interconnected, and the purpose is to solve the problem by replacing traumatic surgery with minimally invasive surgery. Although open traumatic surgery has a good therapeutic effect, this surgery has large trauma, high secondary contamination, will cause serious damage to the patient's body and normal tissues during treatment, and has many postoperative complications, long hospital recovery time, poor recovery and other problems, affecting the quality of life of patients, which will cause heavy economic and psychological burden to patients. Compared with laparotomy, minimally invasive surgery shortens the treatment path, reduces the treatment window, and has the advantages of clear vision, less surgical trauma, faster patient recovery, and shorter hospital stay. With the development of minimally invasive techniques and the popularity of minimally invasive concepts, minimally invasive surgery guided by the concept of path damage control has become the gold standard in the treatment of cardiology, gastroenterology, urology, gastrointestinal surgery, and other diseases. Among them, the effect of minimally invasive surgery on the treatment of liver metastases from colon cancer reflects the advantages of path damage control, reflecting the innovation of the concept and system of disease treatment. Previous radical surgery for liver metastases from colon cancer is often completed by two operations because it requires resection of both organs and is extremely invasive. Although some scholars later advocate one-stage surgery with simultaneous resection, because the anatomical positions of the two organs are too far apart, it is necessary to incise an incision of 40–50 cm in the abdominal wall to complete, with slow postoperative recovery, high incidence rate of complications, and even affecting the progress of comprehensive treatment such as late chemotherapy. With the application and development of laparoscopic technique, not only laparoscopic radical resection of colon cancer has become a routine application, but also laparoscopic technique has been applied in various hepatectomies, thus making one-stage surgery of laparoscopic radical resection of colon cancer combined with resection of liver metastases possible. Minimally invasive surgery for the control of path damage greatly improves the speed of recovery and quality of life of patients after surgery, so that they can better tolerate further treatment.

However, is it correct to blindly pursue path damage control? Can all interventions and treatments be solved by minimally invasive? The answer is certainly no. In addition to the limitations of minimally invasive itself, the first thing we have to consider is the balance between path damage and target damage, and if the target damage is too large, even if the path damage is well controlled, it is unacceptable. Once laparoscopic hepatectomy is performed, if uncontrollable bleeding or surrounding organ damage occurs during the operation, it is best to immediately convert to laparotomy for timely control of the damage. If it is minimally invasive, even if the condition can be finally controlled, it is worth losing, because the target damage caused by minimally invasive surgery has far exceeded its alleviation of path damage.

In addition to minimally invasive surgery, the problem of surgical approach is also an important means of controlling path damage. Selecting the correct surgical approach can not only avoid important blood vessels, nerves, and other tissues and reduce the infestation of normal physiological structures but also strengthen the control ability of intraoperative risks and avoid or reduce the occurrence of intraoperative and postoperative complications. Because the pancreas is located in the retroperitoneum, deep, surrounded by complex blood vessels and nerve distribution, it is particularly important to find a correct and suitable surgical approach for pancreatic surgery. We established individualized pancreatic surgical approaches according to the location, size, number, and nature of different pancreatic lesions, such as the transsplenocolic ligament approach for pancreatic tail lesions, the transomental bursa approach for upper pancreatic lesions, and the retroperitoneoscopic approach for pancreatic back lesions. In particular, the retroperitoneoscopic approach breaks through the conventional thinking, finds another way to avoid entering the peritoneal cavity, thereby reducing the interference with the abdominal organs, can significantly reduce bleeding, pancreatic fistula and other complications, and conducive to the rapid rehabilitation of patients. Moreover, due to the limitation of lacunae and the lack of activated trypsin environment, the retroperitoneoscopic approach also plays a huge role in promoting the treatment of severe pancreatitis and significantly reduces the mortality of severe pancreatitis.

Sometimes a "shortcut" to treatment needs to be found in order to achieve an established intervention effect, what is the "shortcut"? How to find it? For damage control, the shortcut is the shortest path to reduce damage and interference to normal tissues. Laparoscopic hepaticojejunostomy and gastrointestinal anastomosis is well-known that laparoscopic choledochojejunostomy has a narrow operating space and low freedom of operation. If choledochojejunostomy and gastrointestinal anastomosis is to be performed like laparotomy, the intestinal canal needs to be repeatedly flipped, which not only interferes with the normal intestinal peristalsis and easily causes postoperative adhesions but also may cause anteroposterior confusion, resulting in the situation that the direction of anastomosis is opposite from time to time. In a large number of clinical practices, the author found that there were two avascular areas in the mesocolon on both sides of the middle colonic artery, and once the "shortcut" of this avascular area was opened, the jejunum could be directly connected to the upper abdominal space, which the author called the "L-hole" and "R-hole." Through the "R" hole, the jejunum can be directly lifted to the hilum and the region of the head of the pancreas for choledochojejunostomy and pancreaticojejunostomy. Through the "L" hole, the jejunum can be lifted to the left upper quadrant area for gastrointestinal anastomosis. The digestive tract anastomosis through this shortest path has small anastomosis tension, is not easy to angulate, is easy to heal the anastomosis, reduces the occurrence of bile leakage, pancreatic fistula, and gastric emptying disorder, facilitates the operation, and reduces the difficulty of surgical operation. Since the mesocolon will form a fused fascia at the level of the duodenum, opening the "R" hole will directly expose the uncinate process of the pancreas, and if enucleation of the uncinate process tumor of the pancreas is required, it can be operated directly through the "R" hole without the need for Koche incision and mobilization of the duodenum, reducing the effect on normal tissue and structure.

1.4.2 Target Damage Control

Target damage control is to reduce the damage to the target organs, accurately guide, and preserve normal tissue function as much as possible while targeted removal of the lesion. Target damage control is the primary goal to achieve the optimization of intervention means, reflecting the essence of the loss control optimization concept. Such an intervention or treatment cannot be implemented if the target injury is too great and the risk or injury during treatment is unbearable. Achieving target damage control requires precision and refinement of the intervention.

The precision of target damage control is reflected in a comprehensive grasp of the disease system, and precise intervention can be implemented only with a meticulous and in-depth understanding of the intervention goal, which may otherwise lead to severe target damage. In terms of tumor treatment, the previous systemic chemotherapy is ineffective and not well targeted, which can have serious killing effects on normal tissue cells while controlling tumor cells, with great side effects, making it difficult for patients to tolerate. Current cancer treatment has entered the era of precision medicine. Liquid biopsy and genetic detection technology are used to discover the mutated gene targets, find the mechanism and pathway leading to tumorigenesis, invasion and metastasis, and then implement targeted drug therapy to reduce the damage to normal cells while controlling the initiating factors of tumor mutation. This is also the case in the surgical treatment of tumors. With the development of three-dimensional reconstruction and artificial intelligence technology, before surgery, we can not only fully evaluate the location, size, number, and vascular invasion of tumors in combination with imaging data, but also more clearly observe the pipeline distribution and variation around the lesion through three-dimensional image reconstruction, and even plan the most efficient and accurate intervention approach and resection range in advance through artificial intelligence technology. Moreover, intraoperative ultrasound-guided as well as laparoscopic and robotic ICG fluorescence staining and reverse staining techniques make the surgeon more and more intuitive in controlling the intervention goal, which is more convenient for the implementation and promotion of accurate intervention measures.

The refinement of target damage control is reflected in the implementation process of intervention. Fine control and careful operation can reduce the complications and side effects caused by target damage as far as possible. Still taking hepatectomy as an example, the delicate operation is reflected in the control of bleeding and the process of liver dissection, which requires avoiding unnecessary ischemia, bruising and residual nonfunctional areas of the liver as much as possible, and the process of liver dissection should be carefully operated, with ligation or suturing of small vessels or bile duct stumps, and avoiding ligation of large pieces of tissue. At the early stage of the development of liver surgery, Pringle method of total hepatic blood flow occlusion and finger pinching, clamping and liver transection promoted the development of hepatectomy, making it possible to perform extensive resection of the liver. However, extensive blood flow occlusion and liver transection also easily led to the occurrence of postoperative ischemia-reperfusion damage, increasing the risk of postoperative complications such as liver dysfunction, bleeding, bile leakage, and abdominal infection. The comprehensive use of regional hepatic blood flow occlusion technique advocated by us can quickly and finely expose and pre-control the input and output blood flow in the resection area, which can not only effectively control the regional hepatic blood flow but also control the extensive communicating branches between liver segments and the bleeding of hepatic veins, improving the efficiency of blood flow occlusion while avoiding residual hepatic ischemia-reperfusion damage. The continuous development of minimally invasive techniques and surgical instruments, represented by laparoscopy and robotics, has made them more suitable for fine control and operation, allowing them to be gradually applied and promoted in hepatectomy.

1.4.3 Additional Damage Control

An additional damage is a damage that is similar to a side effect or adverse reaction of a drug, that is, a damage that is not compatible with the purpose of the intervention and that causes trauma or side effect to the patient. Additional damage is a secondary damage caused by intervention measures, which is contrary to the concept of risk control. It will not only cause poor prognosis of patients, but also lead to that the intervention measures cannot be further implemented. Therefore, additional damage control is also an important link in damage control, which is related to the quality of intervention means optimization and the patient's tolerance.

At present, the additional damage of therapeutic drugs, that is, adverse reactions, has attracted enough attention of clinical intervention providers, forming a complete set of process for the treatment, observation, follow-up, and reporting of adverse drug reactions and serious adverse reactions, promoting the timely risk control and standardized process of drug treatment. Additional damages in terms of surgical interventions are also a problem that has been afflicting the intervention provider and is a roadblock to the application and promotion of surgical interventions. As far as surgical intervention for severe acute pancreatitis is concerned, the purpose of previous laparotomy is to remove necrotic tissue and infectious foci. However, the trauma caused by surgery is easy to cause the spread of infection, which will bring a second blow to patients and even lead to multiple organ failure. In view of the above problems, we propose the concept of guiding instead of removing and the retroperitoneoscopic surgical approach, the theoretical basis of which is to avoid entering the abdominal cavity to reduce the spread of severe infection, not excessively clean the necrotic tissue to reduce the additional damage to normal tissues, and control the damage within a certain range to reduce the severe systemic reaction. The theory reduces the additional damage of surgical intervention to patients, has high tolerance, and greatly reduces the mortality of severe acute pancreatitis. Tumor-free manipulation in oncologic surgery is also an important measure to control additional damage. Studies have shown that the movement and extrusion of the tumor during surgery is easy to promote the blood dissemination of tumor cells, the direct contact between the tumor and the surrounding tissues will also lead to tumor implantation, and the unresected residual tumor cells are more likely to have tumor recurrence and metastasis. Therefore, we need to follow the "noncontact principle" of malignant tumors during surgery; first of all, preoperative imaging techniques are used to plan the surgical approach and resection plane in advance. The action must be gentle when dissecting the tumor to avoid squeezing the tumor and prevent iatrogenic tumor rupture and dissemination of tumor cells into the blood. If necessary, intraoperative ultrasound and intraoperative navigation techniques are used to accurately locate the tumor to ensure adequate resection margins and achieve R0 resection, and combined vascular resection is also required if the tumor invades the blood vessels. For giant liver cancer, there is not enough operating space, and the anterior approach is feasible when necessary, followed by hepatic blood flow occlusion and parenchymal transection on the affected side, and finally liver mobilization to reduce iatrogenic tumor dissemination caused by tumor extrusion during hepatectomy. Finally, timely removal of the tumor in a sterile specimen bag during minimally invasive surgery and postoperative peritoneal lavage with warm distilled water, chlorhexidine, and fluorouracil are all interventions to prevent the spread and local implantation of cancer cells.

1.5 Significance

The concept of damage control is an important part of the optimization of intervention means, and only by minimizing the damage related to intervention can the purpose of good risk control be achieved. In clinical work, risk control as a countermeasure to cope with the adverse consequences of medical risks is often a double-edged sword, and if it can be properly implemented, the risk can be limited to a controllable state. However, the clinical treatment object is human, the risk of the disease itself, the patient's general condition and the changes during the treatment are difficult to control, and the intervention measures are very likely to cause damage to the intervention goal, intervention path, and surrounding environment, which requires the application of the concept of damage control optimization to achieve the optimal target damage with the least path damage and achieve the best clinical benefit with the least cost of intervention. Damage control breaks the traditional concept of previous implementation of complex intervention for severe patients, greatly changes the management principles for complex and critically ill patients, improves the patient's tolerance while reducing patient trauma, and improves the therapeutic effect.

2 Theoretical Innovation and Optimization

The development and progress of medicine are inseparable from the innovation of theory, which determines the development direction of medicine, and its promotion to the development of medicine far exceeds the progress of technology and equipment. Theory is the summary, refinement, and innovation of practice. Only under the correct theoretical framework can the development of methods and techniques drive medical progress faster.

2.1 Concept

Theoretical innovation refers to the new understanding and foresight of the nature of the disease or treatment, mechanism, and development of the law made by intervention providers in medical practice activities, in view of the new situation and new problems, through rational analysis and exploration. Theoretical innovation is the breakthrough or correction of the original theory and method, and is the exploration and development of the unknown field.

2.2 Characteristics

The formation and development of theoretical system and framework require the promotion of theoretical innovation, and the human understanding of diseases needs to be from superficial to in-depth in continuous theoretical innovation, and the means of treatment and intervention are also from extensive to accurate. Theoretical innovation optimization in medical practice is based on patients as the research object, to obtain better risk control and better intervention means as the research purpose, and theoretical innovation in other disciplines has both commonalities and incompleteness, mainly with the following three characteristics, that is, practicalness, openness, and practicability.

2.2.1 Practicalness

Medicine is a highly practical discipline, and the process of medical practice is both the reality of the theory and the bridge, medium and motivation for the theory to function. Theory comes from practice, and theoretical innovation must also be based on practical innovation. The results of theoretical innovation can also provide theoretical guidance for new practical innovation, and test its correctness and practicability in continuous practice. We need to realize theoretical innovation on the basis of clinical practice, and constantly create and improve new theoretical systems based on new practice, so as to provide scientific guidance for understanding the nature of diseases and advancing the treatment of diseases.

2.2.2 Openness

It is not easy to achieve theoretical innovation. In addition to a large number of practical foundations, it requires an open vision, an inclusive mind and a thinking that keeps abreast of the times. Theoretical innovation requires extensive absorption of the theoretical achievements of predecessors and contemporary scholars, as well as extensive absorption of multidisciplinary theoretical achievements. Existence is reasonable. The current theoretical system through long-term previous development and accumulation will inevitably have the necessity and practicability of existence, but with the rapid development of the times and science and technology, if the theory fails to keep pace with the times, it will lag behind, hinder the progress of the discipline, and sometimes even find that the existing theory runs counter to the reality. At this time, it is required that clinical intervention providers can seek innovation in inheritance, innovation in comparison, and innovation in development so that theoretical innovation can have a solid foundation and keep pace with the times.

2.2.3 Practicability

Medical theory is not a fantasy theory of talking on paper and needs to be repeatedly tested by practice. The fundamental purpose of theoretical innovation lies in the application in practice, and the innovation of medical theory must also come from practice to achieve the unity of practicalness and practicability. Only in this way can the scientific nature and value of theoretical innovation be reflected, otherwise there will be no practical means of intervention under a theoretical system with no practical value, and theoretical innovation without practicality will have no value and meaning of existence.

2.3 Classification

2.3.1 Developmental Theoretical Innovation

Developmental theory innovation is based on affirming and inheriting the original theory, and making new additions and modifications to the original theoretical system and principles according to the development of science and technology and the needs of practice, in order to meet the needs of practical application. Most of the time, the development of new theories is based on the original theory, which is the sublimation of previous experience, as well as the improvement of existing shortcomings. Only by standing on the shoulders of our predecessors can we continuously achieve new breakthroughs and find better solutions to problems.

Typically, theoretical innovations in blood control and hepatic dissection techniques hepatectomy makes liver surgery continue to develop from extensive to refined, and the surgical indications continue to expand to various ranges of the liver. In the primary stage of surgical development, the liver is a forbidden area for surgery, and the development of liver surgery is difficult due to uncontrollable intraoperative bleeding and postoperative complications. With the gradual understanding of the anatomy of the hepatic portal vessels, Pringle pioneered the blood flow occlusion method of the first porta hepatis occlusion, that is, total hepatic blood flow occlusion. Academician Wu Mengchao proposed the normothermic intermittent porta hepatis occlusion method on this basis, combined with the finger pinching and clamping hepatectomy method to carry out hepatectomy, especially a wide range of hepatectomy, promoting the process of liver surgery. However, extensive blood flow blocking and liver transection are more likely to cause postoperative complications such as postoperative liver dysfunction, bile leakage, abdominal infection, etc., which have been unable to meet the treatment needs of doctors and patients. Japanese scholar Makuuchi proposed the theory of anatomical hepatectomy on this basis, that is, systematically remove a liver segment and the area innervated by its portal vein branches together with the artery along the portal vein, including the resection of liver lobe, liver segment, and subliver segment. Under the guidance of the theory of anatomical hepatectomy, the technique of regional blood flow control and anatomical lesion resection of the liver is pushed to a new height using intraoperative ultrasound-guided fine dissection and transection of the liver pedicle and methylene blue staining of the liver segment. Of course, the excessive pursuit of fine liver segment anatomy and resection will also bring about the prolongation of operation time, portal occlusion time, postoperative abnormal liver function, and other complications. In this case, we summarize the anatomical characteristics of hepatic blood flow supply and the characteristics of minimally invasive operation and propose the theory of hepatic blood flow occlusion with "one side and two controls." This theory advocates the comprehensive use of hepatic blood flow occlusion technique to quickly and finely expose and pre-control the input and output blood flow in the resection area. While effectively controlling the regional hepatic blood flow, it can also control the extensive communicating branches between liver segments and the bleeding of hepatic veins, improving the efficiency of blood flow occlusion and liver transection. The theory is based on the affirmation and full understanding of previous theories, combined with the latest advances in anatomical cognition and technology, and summarized and concluded after repeated reflection, selection, and practice. It can be said that compared with the previous theory, this theoretical innovation is more suitable for the current medical environment and treatment needs, but we should recognize that society, medicine, and science and technology are in continuous development and progress, all theories are also in continuous development rather than static, and this hepatic blood flow blocking theory will also be replaced by more effective theories, so recognizing the development attributes of theories can better achieve continuous theoretical innovation and continuously realize the optimization of intervention means.

Associated liver partition and portal vein ligation for staged hepatectomy (ALPPS), proposed by German scholar Hans Schlitt in 2012, is also a theoretical innovation to cope with insufficient residual liver volume after surgery. Before the advent of ALPPS surgery, in order to prevent liver dysfunction after subtotal hepatectomy, preoperative portal vein embolization or portal vein ligation was mainly used to block the portal vein blood flow of the liver segment to be removed, allowing compensatory hyperplasia of the contralateral liver. Due to the slow growth rate of the residual liver volume and the long waiting time for the second surgery, patients tend to lose the best time for surgery due to the progression of the tumor. The ALPPS theory is based on the two-step hepatectomy theory of portal vein blockage, which recognizes the role of the intersegmental traffic branch on the blood supply to the contralateral liver, and aims to increase the blood supply to the preserved side of the liver by surgically blocking the portal vein flow on the side to be resected in the first step and by splitting the liver tissue along the ischemic line. Compared with the traditional two-step hepatectomy with portal vein occlusion, this theoretical method can promote the rapid growth of residual liver volume in the short term, without significantly increasing the surgical risk.

2.3.2 Corrective Theoretical Innovation

Corrective theoretical innovation is based on the needs of medical practice, through repeated induction and summary, to correct or change the long-standing misconceptions and interpretations of relevant theories, in order to achieve better prognosis and promote application. Corrective theoretical innovation is actually achieved on the basis of a full understanding of the original theory. Through practical application, people gradually find that some theories have one or more defects and errors, which mislead the application of methods and techniques under this theoretical system, and even threaten the prognosis and life of patients. This is not a problem of inheritance and development, and it is necessary to sort out its nature and principles and change and revise the overall principle and system.

The treatment of severe acute pancreatitis (SAP) has undergone the change of "early surgery - conservative surgery - extended surgery - reduced surgery - minimally invasive treatment as the lead of comprehensive treatment," which has significantly improved the prognosis of patients with acute severe pancreatitis and reduced the mortality rate through the revised theoretical innovation of changing from "removal-oriented" to "drainage-oriented." SAP is an acute and critical disease with sinister condition, many complications and high mortality, and surgical treatment needs to be selected when the pancreas and peripancreatic necrotic tissue are associated with infection and retroperitoneal abscess. Traditional SAP surgery is mostly based on the removal of the pancreas and surrounding necrotic tissue. This surgical method mostly uses the anterior abdominal wall incision and needs to open the omental bursa, colonic ligament, and pancreatic dorsal membrane. It is easy to cause secondary injury to adjacent organs, so that pancreatic necrotic tissue and infectious secretions inevitably infiltrate into the abdominal cavity, thus aggravating abdominal infection and leading to systemic inflammation. Moreover, the effect of low exudate drainage is poor, which can easily aggravate multiple organ failure such as paralytic intestinal obstruction, intra-abdominal hypertension and even renal insufficiency. Due to the poor surgical effect and high mortality of patients for SAP for a long time, intervention providers began to recognize that the original theory of extended debridement was more likely to exacerbate the secondary effects of inflammation on patients, and that mere improvements to the procedure were no longer able to improve patient prognosis and had to be revised from their theoretical roots. The current intervention providers, through an in-depth understanding of the pathophysiology of pancreatitis, have realized that adequate drainage is the core of the surgical treatment of secondary infection in SAP, and that reasonable and unobstructed drainage is crucial to the success of SAP treatment. Surgical interventions need to follow the principles of minimal invasiveness, simplicity, and effectiveness, and on the basis of proper timing of drainage, choose a modality that is less invasive, easily accessible, easy to manage, and can guarantee the effectiveness of drainage. On this basis, through a profound understanding of the anatomy of the peritoneal cavity around the pancreas and the structure of the retroperitoneal space, we introduced the retroperitoneoscopic technique into the surgical treatment of SAP. The theory innovatively and effectively drains the pancreatic and peripancreatic necrotic tissues along with a large amount of exudate containing a variety of pancreatic-derived digestive enzymes out of the body through the pararenal anterior space in a timely manner, alleviating further edema and necrosis of the pancreatic tissue. The approach is direct, does not interfere with the abdominal cavity, has less surgical trauma, and has smooth drainage. While reducing the infestation of traditional surgery on the abdominal organs and structures, it effectively reduces the complications of enteroparalysis and excessive abdominal pressure, which is conducive to the improvement of the outcome and prognosis of SAP.

Pancreaticojejunostomy is a challenging way of digestive tract reconstruction and an Achilles heel that affects the prognosis of patients after pancreaticoduodenectomy. Pancreatic surgeons have made a variety of attempts over the years in terms of pancreaticojejunostomy modalities and surgical techniques, and so far there is no way of pancreaticojejunostomy that can completely avoid pancreatic fistula. The pancreatic-intestinal anastomosis performed according to the traditional theory of mechanical connection, whether it is a mucosa-to-mucosa lateral anastomosis of the pancreatic duct jejunum, or a sleeve-in, bundled end-lateral anastomosis, is all about the tightness of the anastomosis, and the operation steps are complicated, with more stitches and layers; however, no matter how to improve the technique and steps of the anastomosis, the effect of reducing the incidence of pancreatic fistula after pancreaticoduodenal surgery is not obvious, and it is difficult to solve the occurrence of pancreatic fistula and a series of complications caused by pancreatic fistula. Through repeated thinking on the surgical operation of pancreaticojejunostomy and full understanding of the anatomical healing of pancreaticojejunostomy, we recognize that multi-layer suture seems to be tight, in fact, it is easy to cause ischemia of intestinal wall and pancreatic fracture end. Pancreatic fistula may also occur due to needle damage to the tiny pancreatic duct. In addition, too tight and too dense suture method leads to high anastomotic tension, severe tissue tear caused by suture cutting after tissue edema, which is more likely to lead to the occurrence of pancreatic fistula. Therefore, it is necessary to explore a pancreaticojejunostomy method with the purpose of closely gathering tissue and maintaining anastomotic blood flow, so as to achieve the fastest biological healing with the least mechanical injury. This new theory of pancreaticojejunostomy is a correction of the previous theory to make it more compatible with the physiological healing needs of the anastomosis. Under the guidance of this innovative theory, the author gradually formed the single-layer continuous pancreaticojejunostomy through continuous optimization of the suture method, and initially confirmed the safety and effectiveness of this anastomosis method. Single-layer, wide-needle distance continuous suture of the broken end of the pancreas and the whole layer of jejunal serosa brings the two tissues together without leaving a dead space, which ensures the anastomotic stoma while maintaining the anastomotic strength, and the single-layer continuous suture has less damage to the pancreatic tissue and less anastomotic tension can reduce the tissue suture cutting injury caused by postoperative tissue edema. Under the guidance of the pancreatic duct support tube, the natural approximation between the pancreatic duct mucosa and the jejunal mucosa is completed, so that the pancreatic duct and the jejunal mucosa more easily migrate and grow along the support tube to form a mucosalized natural fistula to form a biological healing. Therefore, while pursuing technological innovation, intervention providers should essentially grasp the main contradiction between intervention means and treatment purposes, timely revise the theory of treatment, and explore a simple, reliable and practical treatment through theoretical innovation.

2.3.3 Autonomous Theoretical Innovation

Autonomous theoretical innovation refers to a new interpretation of anatomical, pathophysiological, or therapeutic issues in the process of medical treatment through an autonomous, new concept, model or theoretical vision in order to better achieve theoretical renewal and thus guide practice. Among them, the more representative one is the rapid rehabilitation surgery theory. This theory, first proposed by Dr. Henrik kehlet of Hvidovre University Hospital, Denmark in 2001, is a complete set of humanized medical theories with the core of reducing surgical stress response and the purpose of promoting safe and rapid recovery of patients. The rapid rehabilitation theory advocates the comprehensive application of various measures that have been confirmed to be effective in the perioperative period to reduce the pathophysiological response of surgery, reduce the incidence of surgical complications and mortality, and promote the accelerated rehabilitation of patients. The rapid rehabilitation theory mainly includes the following three aspects: (1) preoperative patient education, (2) better anesthesia, pain relief, and surgical intervention to reduce surgical stress response, pain, and discomfort; (3) intensive postoperative rehabilitation, including early ambulation and early enteral nutrition. The rapid rehabilitation theory was first applied in cardiac surgery, creatively opened up a safe rehabilitation, cost-effective and high-quality surgical channel, and gradually widely used in orthopedics, urology, gynecology, general surgery, and other disciplines. The autonomous theoretical innovation of rapid rehabilitation better controls the various perioperative stresses of patients, promotes safe recovery rather than just early discharge, and provides safer and more effective medical services while reducing treatment costs, with important social and economic benefits.

"One discovers his ignorance only through learning." Only by recognizing the shortcomings of existing theories can innovative independent theoretical innovations be proposed. At present, the widely recognized Couinaud liver segmentation method is marked by the portal vein into the liver and the hepatic vein out of the liver, which divides the liver into eight natural liver segments. Each liver segment is regarded as an independent functional unit with independent channels for blood supply and blood outflow, and one liver segment is excised with no effect on the surrounding liver segment. However, the author observed many phenomena in the clinical practice of a large number of liver surgical treatments that could not be reasonably explained by the traditional Couinaud segmentation theory, for example, the effect of total hepatic blood flow occlusion during anatomical hemihepatectomy was better than that of simple hemihepatic blood flow occlusion; after hemihepatic vascular transection, the liver parenchyma was not completely ischemic, and some patients' hemihepatic tissues would restore blood supply through potential pathways; in the two-step hepatectomy method, such as simple ligation of the portal vein on the resected side, when the liver parenchyma was not divided, the liver proliferation on the preserved side was slow, and if the liver parenchyma could be split, the compensatory proliferation of the liver on the preserved side was obvious. The author explained the various phenomena of liver blood flow supply by the watershed theory of river flow through irrigation and loss of river water in the region, and found that it seems to be better to describe the blood supply anatomy of the liver by the watershed theory than the traditional Couinaud segmentation method. The river flows through the area and is jointly irrigated by the rivers around the area; the closer to the main trunk of the river, the more water supply is received by the river; the river flow is, the larger the nearby irrigated area is; when one side of the river is intercepted, the supply range of the river will expand to the intercepted side; when the river is intercepted, there will be a short-term water shortage phenomenon in the downstream flow area, and then the intercepted river quickly finds a new outflow channel. The watershed theory of the liver can better explain the changes of liver segmentation in the natural state and the distribution of liver segments during blood flow occlusion. The theory of hepatic blood flow supply based on the watershed theory is a supplement to the traditional liver segmentation theory. Each liver region is not independent but supplied by the surrounding liver pedicle, and the adjacent hepatic veins flow out together. The "watershed theory" of liver anatomy is expected to change the theoretical basis of the whole liver surgery and bring new changes to the intraoperative blood control technique of the liver, the technique of liver transection, and the radical cure method of malignant tumors.

2.4 Significance

Theory comes from practice and is higher than practice, and at the same time, it can react to practice and guide practice. While creating more and more valuable achievements for society, theoretical innovation can also enrich and improve people's knowledge and theoretical structure and ability with the times, and promote the continuous development and progress of society. In clinical practice, intervention providers need to solve the theoretical problems faced in the current medical development and solve the problems of improving the ability to promote health and prevent and treat diseases. Theory plays a role in cognition, explaining phenomena, guiding practice, and solving problems, of which practice and application are more valuable. Clinical intervention providers should not indulge in the existing medical theoretical basis and model, but fully recognize the great driving effect that theoretical innovation can bring, continuously lead the innovative application of technology, and improve the ability to solve practical problems. In actual clinical work, through the development, revision, and independent innovation of the original theory, the author makes the theory more consistent with objective laws and stronger guidance for clinical practice, so that conventional clinical intervention methods are continuously optimized, difficult and complicated diseases are effectively diagnosed and treated, and patients' needs are fully satisfied, thus promoting the leapfrog improvement of the level of clinical treatment activities and medical quality.

3 Path Module Optimization

Due to the differences in the overall medical conditions, technical level, and patient distribution of hospitals at all levels in China, we often find that there will be very different changes in a diagnosis and treatment plan or treatment means during the specific implementation process in clinical practice, which may be formal or qualitative. Especially in some complex intervention processes, it is possible that the forms and steps of intervention will be missed, and it is also possible that the predetermined requirements may not be met in the quality of completion, which will affect the promotion and application of new technologies and new businesses on the one hand, and will also cause imbalance in the medical level on the other hand. If at the early stage of application and development, we can establish a path-based and patterned method to simplify and proceduralize the complex intervention process, which can not only shorten the process of learning, more quickly and effectively master this technology and skill, but also standardize various indicators and ensure the standardization and unification of quality.

3.1 Concept

Path patterning is to simplify the operation process into fixed and unified paths and patterns according to core functions or separate multiple modules with standard forms according to functional blocks. Pathing and patterning is a form of simplification and a form of standardization, not simplicity for simplicity's sake, nor omission for standardization's sake. Pathing and patterning optimization is based on the intervention provider's full understanding of the intervention and repeated thinking summary, and is an accurate grasp of the key nodes in the intervention process, as well as a high degree of condensation of the key steps. Pathing and patterning are not static, need to be continuously tested, supplemented and improved in continuous practical applications, and also need to be not updated and advanced with the development of medical concepts and technologies.

3.2 Characteristics

1. Proceduralization: Pathing and patterning are summarizing seemingly complex programs into a set of programs with fixed formats. Through these procedures, intervention providers can be familiar with and implement specific measures of intervention, avoid the waste of time and resources caused by beginners who cannot grasp the key points, and improve medical efficiency as much as possible. The clinical path we use in the face of a disease in clinical practice is actually the embodiment of proceduralization. By summarizing the medical intervention process into a series of procedural steps or operating processes, it is convenient to implement it under different medical environments and conditions.

2. Standardization: Different treatment plans or measures may be used in different regions, hospitals, and individuals in the face of the same disease, and even the deviation of implementation quality may occur in the specific implementation process of the same treatment plan. The pathing and patterning optimization can standardize medical behaviors, uniformly implement standards, avoid the arbitrariness of medical behaviors, help to improve the quality of medical treatment, eliminate potential medical safety hazards, and reduce the occurrence of medical errors or accidents. After pathing and patterning optimization, the intervention measures become easier to implement and more rule-based, and the level of different physicians has less effect on the medical effect, which can reduce the diagnosis and treatment differences, avoid the arbitrariness of treatment, and improve the homogeneity.
3. Efficiency: The proposal of pathing and patterning is ultimately for clinical application and solving practical clinical problems. Pathing and patterning optimization is the result of long-term thinking and summary by experts in various disciplines, and is the condensation and induction of a large number of clinical experiences. On the one hand, it can reduce the waste of resources and reduce medical costs, and on the other hand, it can improve the quality of diagnosis and treatment and improve the implementation efficiency.

3.3 Classification

3.3.1 Pathing of Clinical Diagnosis and Treatment

The clinical path that is now widely implemented in clinical practice is the embodiment of pathing and patterning optimization. The clinical path emerged in the United States in the mid-1980s and became a standardized management model for clinical medicine commonly used in the United States in the early 1990s. Because the clinical path can not only implement the key quality management principles but also save social resources, it has been rapidly promoted and used in many countries and regions. The clinical path refers to a medical and nursing standard with strict working procedures and accurate time requirements jointly formulated by a group of personnel in the hospital for the monitoring, treatment, rehabilitation, and nursing of a certain disease, in order to reduce the delay of rehabilitation and waste of resources and achieve the purpose of optimizing the benefits of medical quality. The clinical path is generally developed for a specific group of diseases or operations. In the process of developing them, it is necessary to integrate the knowledge of multiple disciplines such as clinical, anesthesia, pharmacy, testing, nursing, nutrition, rehabilitation, psychology, hospital management, and even law and ethics, based on the information of treatment, care, auxiliary examination, laboratory tests, medication, common complications, and medical costs of patients with the disease in our hospital, and to use the concept of evidence-based medicine, so that they can be combined with the latest advances in medical and nursing care of the disease reported at home and abroad. The final formation of clinical path needs to go through the process of preparation and formulation, and is continuously improved and optimized in the implementation, improvement, monitoring, and evaluation, so that its content is more comprehensive, the project is more reasonable, and more in line with the actual work of the undergraduate department.

The establishment of clinical path can not only standardize the treatment plan and medical procedures, reduce the individual differences between different intervention providers, and improve the efficiency and quality of treatment but also reduce some unnecessary and unreasonable treatment behaviors, effectively reduce medical costs and rationalize the use of health resources; and by setting the time to complete each step, it can shorten the hospitalization time, save treatment costs, and enhance the planning of treatment activities. The clinical path is a standardized treatment model that can regulate medical behavior, reduce socioeconomic costs, and contribute to the improvement of medical quality through continuous monitoring and regular evaluation. The clinical path also provides a working mode of multiprofessional collaboration to ensure that the expected therapeutic effect is achieved within the established time while the disciplines are reasonably configured, prompting the effective use of medical resources. In the implementation process of clinical path, patients and their families can also understand the process and time arrangement of diagnosis and treatment implementation, facilitating the affected party to better understand and cooperate with the diagnosis and treatment work of the hospital, promoting the communication and communication between doctors and patients, and improving the patient's satisfaction.

3.3.2 Standardization of Auxiliary Operation

At present, minimally invasive surgery including laparoscopy and robotics has become the direction of surgical development, of which Trocar arrangement is the first step of surgery and the key factor to determine whether the surgery is smooth or even successful. If the Trocar arrangement is unreasonable, it will not only affect the smoothness of the operation, affecting the dissection suturing and knotting operations, but also easily cause the fatigue of the surgeon, making it difficult to maintain attention and stable surgical operations for a long time. Serious irrationality will also lead to difficulty in tumor exposure, uncontrollable bleeding, collateral damage to the surrounding organs, and then conversion to laparotomy, and even endanger the life safety of patients. However, the Trocar arrangement is different for different procedures. The patient's height, weight and tumor anatomical position will affect the distribution of trocar foramen. If a simple, easy to learn and patterned Trocar arrangement method can be summarized according to different conditions, most surgical requirements can be covered through minor adjustment, which can play a huge role in promoting the minimally invasive process of surgical operation.

Currently, the majority of primary care hospitals lack experience in minimally invasive surgery, and even if the surgeon is already proficient in performing the relevant open procedure, once laparoscopic surgery needs to be attempted, the Trocar arrangement will be a decisive factor in determining whether the surgery can be performed successfully. In terms of Trocar arrangement, many beginners will learn the surgical atlas and tutorials and study the surgical videos of large centers. However, on the one hand, the atlases and tutorials tend to focus on the surgical approach and technique, and most of them do not focus on the Trocar arrangement. On the other hand, the major centers often have their own habits and experiences in the Trocar arrangement, and have not summarized a set of principles and patterns of Trocar arrangement that are simple, easy to learn, and can be widely promoted. In view of the author's understanding of the importance of trocar arrangement and the experience in large-sample laparoscopic and robotic hepatobiliary and pancreatic surgery, the author continuously optimized the Trocar arrangement in combination with the intraoperative operation experience and the problems encountered, and summarized the patterned hole layout method, which has a significant effect on improving the operation comfort, improving the operation efficiency, and reducing the conversion rate. The author's patterned hole arrangement method follows the four major hole arrangement principles, namely, the principle of umbilical perimeter main operation lateral mirror, the principle of main line symmetry, the principle of traction, and the principle of flat abdomen 8 cm spacing. There are corresponding patterned holes for all common procedures. Through the optimization of Trocar arrangement mode, it is convenient for beginners to learn from it, there are rules to follow, it can avoid the occurrence of serious errors to improve the safety of surgery, and the patterned hole layout method is convenient for promotion and application, it can effectively shorten the learning curve, improve the operation comfort, reduce the difficulty of surgery, shorten the operation time, not only can improve the prognosis of patients but also can promote the minimally invasive promotion and popularization of surgery.

3.3.3 Patterning of Intervention Means

Laparoscopic hepatectomy is still considered difficult and more dangerous than traditional open hepatectomy because of the complex liver anatomy, rich blood supply, deep anatomical location of some liver segments, difficulty in laparoscopic vascular block of the hilar region, and difficulty in intraoperative hemostasis. In recent years, with the application of endoscopic cutter stapler in laparoscopic liver surgery, rapid and effective liver tissue transection has become possible. Through summarizing the vascular anatomical distribution of the left lateral lobe of the liver, the characteristics of laparoscopic surgery, and the experience in the use of linear cutter stapler, the author took the lead in proposing the concept of laparoscopic patterned left lateral lobectomy of the liver, and proposed a standardized and patterned process for the surgical steps and the use of related devices. Aiming at the difficulty in traditional laparoscope-guided anatomy and treatment of segment II and III hepatic vessels as well as left hepatic vein, this patterned left lateral lobectomy method puts forward the programmed and standardized methods of not anatomizing extrahepatic vessels, thinning hepatic parenchyma with harmonic scalpel and linear cutter stapler transection. This patterned surgical method does not require hepatic portal occlusion to reduce intraoperative bleeding, can effectively avoid hepatic ischemia-reperfusion injury and gastrointestinal congestion and edema caused by hepatic portal occlusion, and promote the rapid recovery of patients. Compared with laparoscopic traditional left lateral lobectomy, the intraoperative blood loss is significantly reduced, and the overall medical costs are not significantly increased. Due to its simple steps and relatively low technical requirements, junior surgeons can also quickly master it. Through the optimization of the mode of laparoscopic left lateral lobectomy, the surgical process is simpler, faster, more prominent, with high safety and reliability. Its normalized and standardized operation procedure is easy for beginners and primary hospitals to learn, carry out and promote, and gradually becomes the "standard" procedure for left external hepatic lobectomy.

3.3.4 Modularization of Complex Operations

For complex surgeries, many surgical steps and high difficulty in operation are the main reasons affecting the quality of surgery, and often such surgeries can only be completed in large surgical centers and are difficult to carry out in general hospitals. If the complex surgical steps can be split into modules like building blocks, proceduralized operation modes can be formed in their respective modules, and the complex surgery can be simplified, perhaps more hospitals and doctors can master the standardized process and surgical skills of complex surgery. Since laparoscopic radical gastrectomy for gastric cancer lacks overall vision and the surgeon loses the accurate tactile sensation of the hand, these put forward higher requirements for the surgeon's anatomical understanding and minimally invasive operating skills. On the basis of fully understanding a series of problems such as perigastric anatomical space, anatomical location and vascular variation, and repeatedly thinking about the surgical operation process, some scholars have proposed the surgical mode of modular laparoscopic radical gastrectomy for gastric cancer, attributed the complex operation to be completed during the operation to different modules such as surgical position, Trocar layout, perigastric tissue mobilization, and lymph node dissection, and performed the surgical operation in an orderly manner according to the process, so as to achieve clear objectives, prominent focus, and targeted. By modularizing the surgical procedure, on the one hand, the modular decomposition is conducive to deepening the surgeon's understanding of laparoscopic lower abdominal regional anatomy and understanding of the surgical process, on the other hand, following the long-term study and summarized surgical steps can reduce the interference and damage to the normal tissue structure during the early exploration, not only accelerate the surgical process, make the surgical process more smooth, but also have a lower incidence of postoperative complications, faster recovery can better tolerate the comprehensive treatment of tumors, and improve the quality of life and prognosis of patients to a certain extent. In addition, a series of convenient and reasonable anatomical approaches and simple, coherent, and efficient surgical procedures summarized under the modular theory reduce the difficulty of surgery, shorten the learning curve of surgeons, reduce the running-in process between surgeons and assistants, bring important clinical benefits to the majority of patients, and can produce good socioeconomic value through the simplification of surgical procedures and the summary of technical routes.

3.4 Steps

3.4.1 Clinical Practice

All theories are derived from practice, and this is especially true of medicine as a practical science. In order to summarize the path from the specific operation, summarize the mode and divide it into modules, it must go through a large number of clinical practices and need to touch and scroll in clinical practice for a long time in order to find the problem and propose the method to solve the problem. Without the test of clinical practice, intervention providers cannot realize the advantages and disadvantages of various interventions and diagnosis and treatment methods and cannot find the key crux affecting clinical operation and patient prognosis. With the modularity of laparoscopic radical gastrectomy for gastric cancer, beginners in the learning curve often aim to be able to complete the standard radical surgery. Due to the lack of experience in the operation, there are still few accidents encountered during the operation, and the lack of experience in the specific operation steps, it is natural that the optimization methods of patterning and modularity cannot be proposed. Only after a large number of surgical operations can the defects and shortcomings of the original theories and methods be discovered, and only then can the modular form and process be simplified and generalized, and the progress and development of medicine be promoted.

3.4.2 Generalization and Summarization

The generalization and summarization after a lot of practice is actually the process from quantitative change to qualitative change. Practice is the process of accumulating quantitative change, and generalization and summarization is the catalyst of qualitative change. In clinical practice, practice alone is not enough, and if practice is no longer generalized, not summarized, and refined, it cannot be elevated to theory, and such doctors are at best skilled workers or cutters, not only cannot break through the bottleneck of self-technical ability but also cannot use their own experience as a booster for common progress in this field. Taking the Trocar arrangement problem of minimally invasive surgery as example, because each patient is unique, it is impossible to have the same tumor location and the same body size. Therefore, no matter how many surgeries have been done, it is impossible to achieve a reasonable layout when encountering new problems. This requires that in practice, according to the specific experience of each operation, according to the opinions and suggestions of different surgeons on Trocar hole, according to their own understanding and thinking on the hole problem, the patterned hole method suitable for different patient sizes and tumor positions is summarized and summarized, so that the previous hole method according to the anatomical position of the body surface no longer meets the requirements of individualized minimally invasive surgery.

3.4.3 Practical Application

Theory comes from practice and needs to go to practice, the final foothold or practical application. Whether it is a large number of clinical practices or long-term thinking summary, in the final analysis, it is to improve the level of diagnosis and treatment, in order to promote the overall development of medical backward areas. We should achieve the unification of theory and practice in clinical practice, not as a "theorist," but as a "practitioner." If it is not tested and polished by practice, the best experience and theory cannot prove its superiority, much less be recognized by the peers of this profession, and can only remain on paper. After summarizing and proposing the theory of patterned two-step laparoscopic left lateral lobectomy, the author immediately carried out this technical method in a comprehensive manner in this department. After demonstrating its safety and effectiveness, it has been widely popularized in national conferences and various training courses, and studied and applied by hospitals at all levels nationwide. At present, this method has become the standard for left lateral lobectomy.

3.5 Significance

Pathing and patterning optimization is the generalization and sublimation of intervention means, which is based on a large number of long-term practice and in-depth thinking summary, and is of great significance for simplifying the medical process, standardizing medical behavior, and improving the quality of medical care. After condensing the complex diagnosis and treatment process and intervention means into the paths, modes, and modules with clear logic, reasonable structure, and smooth procedure, the intervention provider can more easily understand the focus of the whole treatment process and better grasp the key nodes of the intervention measures, which is conducive to shortening the process of learning curve and simplifying the complex operation. In addition, after the implementation of pathing and patterning, all operating means and processes have rules to follow, which are more reasonable and standardized, reducing the impact of different clinical experience and medical conditions on the quality of medical treatment, reducing the differences in the implementation of diagnosis and treatment process by medical institutions at all levels, improving the overall medical level, which is not only conducive to the implementation of tiered diagnosis and treatment but also can solve the social problem of "difficulty in seeing a doctor" in China to a certain extent.

4 Cost-Benefit Optimization

With the development of medical science and technology, we have more and more advanced tools for disease detection and treatment, but with this comes more and more expensive medical care. The rapid rise of medical costs has become the main reason restricting people to enjoy advanced medical technology achievements, and is also the main contradiction that leads to the social problem of "difficult and expensive medical treatment" in China, which has become an urgent problem to be solved in the field of medical and health care in China. Medical resources, especially quality medical resources, are limited and cannot meet the unlimited medical needs of people, nor can they meet the medical needs of everyone. In the actual medical process, we always face difficult choices when making decisions. This section describes how to optimize interventions by analyzing and comparing costs and benefits for different diagnosis and treatment options.

4.1 Concept

Cost-benefit optimization is based on medical theory, by measuring and describing medical costs and results in a monetized form, to select or optimize safe and effective interventions or combinations with better economic effects. It emphasizes not only the maximum effectiveness of interventions but also the economic affordability of patients and society.

In the previous treatment, intervention providers often pay attention to emphasizing the safety and effectiveness of drugs or treatments and ignore the economic problems, which leads to increased medical costs, waste of health resources, and increased economic burden on patients and society. The purpose of our proposed concept of intervention optimization is to achieve the best prognosis effect, emphasizing that in the medical process, it reduces the harm to patients, reduces the consumption of resources, and seeks to meet the interests of most people as much as possible in the allocation of medical resources. The optimization of cost-benefit emphasizes the economy of intervention. It does not mean to use simple, inexpensive tests and treatments, nor does it deny the progress and efficiency brought by advanced medical treatments. Instead optimization can achieve the best results with the least amount of medical costs and resources. Cost-benefit optimization can avoid excessive waste of medical resources and funds and reduce the economic burden on patients and society.

4.2 Necessity

Medical resources are limited and people's pursuit of life and medical quality is unlimited, so in the process of medical treatment, it is necessary to realize the reasonable distribution of medical resources, avoid the waste of medical resources, and maximize the utilization efficiency of medical resources. In order to achieve a rational allocation of medical resources, it is necessary to set a definite limit for the use of medical resources, and to have a clear plan and determination of when and what resources are to be used for what disease conditions, rather than to use them blindly and wastefully. Realistic medical conditions cannot meet all medical needs or preferences. Social and personal wealth is limited, and excessive spending on medical care is at the expense of giving up other valuable materials and services. For example, PET-CT has the advantages that other examinations do not have in the judgment of benign and malignant tumors, and the sensitivity and specificity of diagnosis are high. We often encounter the situation that PET-CT is actively required during routine physical examination in clinical practice. Although PET-CT examination plays a certain role in tumor screening, there is still a more direct and economical examination method as a physical examination, and the high examination cost of PET-CT will not only increase the economic burden of patients but also encroach on the medical resources of patients who must undergo PET-CT examination, resulting in dual resource waste.

Under the past price distribution system, as long as someone pays the cost, no matter whether it is necessary and effective, any possible diagnosis and treatment means can be provided, but this inefficient diagnosis and treatment method will cause great waste of medical resources. Cost-benefit optimization adds the consideration of economic costs on the basis of ensuring the prognostic benefits. While improving the diagnosis and treatment technology and optimizing the means of intervention, the cost of medical measures and the benefits obtained are compared. Through the control of diagnosis and treatment costs, the limited resources are used in the areas with the best effect. The direction, order, and combination of distribution are determined through cost-benefit optimization to further improve the utilization rate of medical resources.

4.3 Specific Strategies

Medical resource allocation should try to avoid waste and consider the maximization of patient and social interests. In the decision and practice of specific medical measures, it is necessary to compare and evaluate the benefits obtained and the costs incurred, which include not only economic but also non-economic factors, and to determine the final solution through a cost-benefit analysis of the proposed solution based on a comprehensive analysis of the costs paid and the benefits obtained. Cost-benefit optimization in this section investigates benefits in a broad sense rather than monetization benefits in a narrow sense, and intervention providers need to optimize control costs on the basis of comprehensive consideration of effects, utilities, and monetization benefits.

The specific operation steps to implement cost-benefit optimization include the following points: first, it is necessary to clarify the cost required by each project; second, it is necessary to determine all the benefits obtained by implementing the project; third, it is necessary to quantify the cost and benefits of the project; and finally, it is necessary to carry out reasonable analysis and evaluation on the cost and benefits of the expected investment.

4.3.1 Cost-Effective Analysis (CEA)

Cost-effective analysis refers to an analysis method that the economic efficiency of the evaluated intervention program is expressed by the cost/effectiveness ratio, and the cost and effectiveness indicators of the evaluation program are analyzed and compared by comparing the effect size achieved by the unit cost invested by each program. The effectiveness here is expressed directly as a clinical outcome indicator after the administration of the intervention, which can be divided into an intermediate indicator and an endpoint indicator. Intermediate indicators refer to the observation indicators indirectly reflecting the clinical results, such as blood pressure, blood glucose, and other biochemical indicators. Endpoint indicators refer to the results directly reflecting the treatment and prognosis, such as morbidity, survival rate, and mortality.

The guiding ideology of cost-effective analysis method is to achieve the determined treatment goal at the lowest cost or the maximum diagnosis and treatment effect that should be obtained by consuming certain medical resources, which is generally used for the comparison of different plans with the same goal and similar indicators. In theory, the cost is the same or similar among the programs, and the program with better effectiveness is selected. When the effectiveness is the same or similar, the program with lower cost should be selected. For example, when robots are applied to radical prostatectomy surgery, it is often questionable whether expensive robotic equipment will increase the burden on patients and whether patients can benefit from advanced technology. By analyzing the cost-effectiveness of robotic surgery and laparotomy, we found that despite the higher cost of robotic surgery, robotic surgery has faster operative time, less intraoperative bleeding, faster postoperative recovery, and no significant difference in postoperative morbidity and survival compared with laparotomy. Moreover, because patients have a short postoperative hospital stay and robotic surgery does not bring more burden to patients in terms of overall treatment costs, it can be considered that robotic radical prostatectomy can be the most optimal treatment after comprehensive analysis.

4.3.2 Cost-Utility Analysis (CUA)

Cost-utility analysis is the calculation of the ratio of the incremental cost derived from a program to the incremental health benefit attributable to the program, which is often used in the quality assessment of treatment options for nonfatal health outcomes. In cost-benefit optimization, the benefit of treatment is not measured by traditional indicators such as simple morbidity and mortality, but by measuring quality of life and years of life, which requires the use of health measurement methods such as Quality-Adjusted Life Years (QALYs). QALYs is the mathematical product of life expectancy and the mass of the remaining life years (QALYs = ΣMi = 1qiTi), with 1 year of complete physical health equal to 1 quality-adjusted life year and death equal to 0 adjusted life years. QALYs focus on both the length and quality of life and can evaluate the cost-utility of treatment regimens by obtaining the cost required for 1 quality-adjusted life-year. Many countries judge the cost-effectiveness of health care measures by assessing the investment required to add 1 quality-adjusted life year to determine whether they are covered by insurance. The standard value is generally based on the GDP of various countries. For example, the United States generally takes the investment of 50,000 US dollars required for adding 1 quality-adjusted life year as the standard, and no more than 50,000 US dollars is considered to have good cost-effectiveness; the United Kingdom and Australia mostly use 27,000 US dollars/QALY as the standard; China generally uses 11,900 US dollars/QALY as the standard.

For example, hypertension, a common chronic disease, has become the first major disease in China and the primary disease burden for Chinese residents. The choice of its quality program is not only a medical problem but also an important issue in health economics. Previous medical guidelines have recommended drugs and treatments primarily to assess their efficacy, with little attention to the costs and benefits of treatment. The cost of hypertension drug treatment mainly includes the cost of drug purchase, the cost of follow-up visit for patients, and the treatment cost when the drug side effects occur. The benefits are mainly reflected in that antihypertensive treatment is used to avoid cardiovascular and cerebrovascular diseases in some patients, improve the quality of life and prolong the life span, thereby saving the cost of treating these cases. When applying the quality-adjusted life-year approach, the cost required to obtain one life-year with quality of life needs to be analyzed and then compared with standard values to evaluate the cost-effectiveness of medical interventions. The selection of hypertension treatment plan needs to pay attention to cost-utility assessment and analysis and optimal selection to prevent the waste of resources caused by excessive treatment and to maximize the limited medical and health resources.

4.3.3 Cost-Benefit Analysis (CBA)

Cost-benefit analysis refers to a method to compare, analyze, and evaluate the monetary value of all expected benefits and expected costs of various options under the condition of scarce medical resources, which is used as a reference and basis for the selection and decision-making of intervention providers. Cost-benefit analysis needs to evaluate the advantages and disadvantages of each diagnosis and treatment plan with monetary value when the benefits can be measured with monetary value. Since the results of costs and benefits are displayed with monetary value, it can be used not only for the comparison of different plans for the same disease but also for the comparison of different plans for multiple diseases. It should be noted that cost-benefit analysis is only suitable for describing the benefit with monetary value. When the results are not suitable for conversion to monetary amount, such as quality of life or satisfaction, which is difficult to quantify, this analysis method is difficult to apply. The use of cost-benefit analysis in the medical field is often focused on antimicrobial use and vaccination. For example, the cost-benefit analysis of different antibacterial drugs in the treatment of severe infections is performed by calculating the monetary value of all costs and final therapeutic effects such as drugs, treatment, follow-up, and missed work, and obtaining the benefit-cost ratio of each drug in order to select the optimal antibacterial drug regimen.

4.4 Significance

In all aspects of social life, people always want to get the best results for the cost they pay, or to get similar results at the lowest cost, and this is especially true in the medical field. Life is invaluable, but medical resources are limited. Making full use of limited medical resources to maximize the benefits of patients and society requires the use of cost-benefit analysis to achieve the effective distribution of medical resources through the optimization of diagnosis and treatment behaviors and intervention means.

1. In today's booming development of medical science and technology, new basic theories, diagnostic methods, therapeutic drugs, technologies, and devices emerge endlessly, and it is difficult for intervention providers to quickly and deeply understand, and when facing sudden new technologies and new methods, they often do not know how to choose. It is better to combine the latest medical progress with actual clinical work, and sometimes there is an irrational use of excessive medical treatment, which may cause the occurrence of new adverse events on the one hand and also aggravate the economic burden of patients on the other hand, resulting in the waste of medical resources. Through cost-benefit analysis, intervention providers can fully understand the costs and possible effects of various examination and treatment methods in the implementation process, in order to make a more rapid judgment, selection, and optimization and develop the corresponding intervention means and program combination according to the patient's condition, possible risks, and optional intervention means.
2. The most advanced diagnosis and treatment methods will certainly promote the progress of various professional fields, but the ensuing high economic costs will also bring heavy burden to individuals and society. The optimization of interventions that we have described in previous chapters focuses on safety and effectiveness and on how to achieve maximum treatment effects with minimal damage without taking into account the economy of interventions. Due to the economic and social nature of human beings, the economic burden that each person can bear is different. The economic factors of the interventions need to be considered in the treatment and the impact on the patient, and not the most advanced and effective means are the most appropriate and reasonable. The cost-benefit optimization in this section is to scientifically and rationally analyze the cost-effectiveness of different intervention means for the same disease on the basis of ensuring the safety and effectiveness of the diagnosis and treatment process, analyze and evaluate its economic value, optimize the allocation of intervention means from controllable root causes, and finally select the best intervention means that are easy to use, have a positive effect, and have a reasonable price. Cost-benefit optimization can not only help hospitals effectively control medical costs and make the selection of clinical decisions more optimized but also further reduce the economic burden borne by patients and select appropriate intervention means according to the economic capacity of patients in order to rationally utilize and distribute medical resources and effectively reduce the phenomenon of resource waste.
3. Current intervention providers often flock to new diagnostic methods, new therapeutic drugs, and new surgical methods, and at many times are in the stage of blindly following the trend, regardless of their own medical level and the economic situation of patients. Such a medical model is prone to excessive medical treatment. For example, PET-CT is recommended for benign and malignant tumors that can be confirmed by MRI; whole-exon examination is recommended for tumor patients with genetic mutations that can be judged by immunohistochemistry; high-grade drugs are used for chronic diseases that can be controlled by taking conventional drugs; robotic surgery is performed for gallstones that

can be solved by laparoscopic surgery, and the above and other conditions are excessive application of new interventions. Adequate use of cost-benefit optimization in the medical field not only allows for strong economic control of all medical practices but also promotes the rationalization and optimal allocation of interventions and medical resources, and enhances the use of medical resources while transforming medical work patterns into economic control.

In summary, the role that cost-benefit analysis plays in healthcare has started to become increasingly important. Through cost-benefit analysis, it can not only help clinical intervention providers to timely and comprehensively master the implementation of various diagnosis and treatment measures, effectively control costs, save medical resources, reduce the economic pressure on patients and society to seek medical treatment but also help intervention providers to effectively select and optimize the intervention means with higher cost-effectiveness ratio, improve the overall medical ability, and facilitate the development of health services in China. It is undesirable to ignore the cost of treatment and only consider its safety and efficacy, and it is not possible to do real and permanent medical risk control. We must keep abreast of the times in the daily treatment process, and strictly combine the economic and social costs and benefits at this stage to optimize the cost-effectiveness of all aspects of the treatment process.

5 Application of Artificial Intelligence

With the rapid development of health informatization and the wide application of medical big data, artificial intelligence technology has become a new trend of medical information technology exhibition, has been widely tried and applied in intelligent imaging, intelligent pathology, intelligent clinical decision-making, and other aspects, and is expected to become a technology that can be popularized and promoted in the field of surgery. Artificial intelligence has a huge development prospect in health management, drug research and development, disease diagnosis and treatment, precision medicine, and other aspects, and is expected to play an important role in reducing medical costs, improving the efficiency and rationality of diagnosis and treatment, and improving the uneven allocation of medical resources. With the development of artificial intelligence rising to a national strategy, our clinical intervention providers need to change their working concept, learn intelligent technology, standardize medical behavior, and encourage cooperation to comply with the opportunities and challenges brought to us by artificial intelligence medical treatment.

5.1 Concept

Artificial intelligence (AI) is a new technical science that studies the theory, method, technology, and application used to simulate, extend, and expand human intelligence, and its purpose is to use computers to simulate human thinking processes and intelligent behaviors (such as learning, reasoning, thinking, planning). Artificial intelligence is a highly integrated interdisciplinary discipline, which is the product of research based on various disciplines such as computer science, cybernetics, information theory, neuropsychology, philosophy, and linguistics, and its research contents mainly include natural language understanding, machine learning and knowledge acquisition, knowledge processing systems, computer vision, automatic reasoning, search methods, intelligent robots, automatic program design, and expert systems. AI is gradually emerging as a strong impetus to subvert various fields. Through the application of AI in medical institutions, it can improve the production efficiency of hospitals, enhance the service level of primary care, play the advantages of AI in the diagnosis, prediction, treatment, and management services of diseases, and help improve the uncertainty of surgical treatment and the imbalance of surgical level development.

5.2 Development of Artificial Intelligence

The history of artificial intelligence dates back to the 1950s, and the concept of artificial intelligence was first proposed by computer scientist John McCarthy at the first artificial intelligence seminar held at Dartmouth University in the United States in 1956, marking the birth of the artificial intelligence discipline. After more than 60 years of development, especially in the past 10 years, with the rapid improvement of algorithms and computing capacity, driven by new theories and technologies such as Internet, big data, supercomputing, sensing network and economic and social development needs, artificial intelligence technology has undergone revolutionary development, showing new functions such as deep learning, integration, human-computer coordination, and independent manipulation, which has profoundly changed human life.

At present, artificial intelligence has become a new focus of international competition, a new engine of economic development, and a new opportunity for social construction. Europe, the United States, and other countries have issued plans to promote the development of artificial intelligence from the national level. In 2016, the United States government released the Report on the National Strategic Plan for Artificial Intelligence Research and Development, and in December 2016, the United Kingdom also released the Strategic Report on Artificial Intelligence, advocating the development of artificial intelligence to improve enterprise competitiveness, government governance capacity, and comprehensive national strength. In May 2016, China issued the Implementation Plan for the Three-year Action of "Internet +" Artificial Intelligence. In July 2017, the State Council pointed out in the Development Plan for the New Generation of Artificial Intelligence that the application of artificial intelligence in the field of intelligent medical treatment should be deepened, new models and means of artificial intelligence diagnosis and treatment should be popularized and applied, and a rapid and accurate intelligent medical system should be established. The kick-off meeting of "New Generation Artificial

Intelligence Development Plan and Major Science and Technology Project" was held in Beijing in November 2017, which marks that the development of artificial intelligence in China has entered the stage of comprehensive kick-off and implementation.

5.3 Application of Artificial Intelligence in Medicine

Artificial intelligence technology based on medical information big data provides a more convenient and optimized way for medical services. The application of artificial intelligence in the medical field not only brings about the innovation of medical technology but also promotes the transformation of the whole medical diagnosis and treatment model and plays a huge role in promoting the traditional human-led clinical decision-making.

At present, the research on the use of artificial intelligence technology for disease diagnosis and treatment mainly focuses on the following two aspects: firstly, through intelligent analysis of data, images, audio, video, and other medical image data, accurately extract the characteristics of the disease, draw cognitive conclusions on the pathophysiological changes of patients, which is helpful for faster and more accurate prevention and diagnosis of diseases. Secondly, using artificial intelligence to quickly read massive medical literature, case data, and diagnosis and treatment plan, quickly extract key information from a large number of fragmented data, through reasoning, analysis, comparison, induction, and summary, and carry out intelligent auxiliary clinical decision-making and other issues of research.

5.3.1 Impact on Disease Diagnostic Patterns

Artificial intelligence is now playing an increasingly prominent role in medical image recognition, with its superior cognitive abilities compensating for the lack of time and experience of the intervention providers. Traditional medical imaging research based on machine learning works around the image characteristics specified by the intervention providers, which makes the model only judge around the semi-quantitative information of the specified characteristics, resulting in the weak generalization ability of the model and classifying the degree of disease development. Artificial intelligence-assisted diagnosis and treatment based on big data intelligent technology is based on standardized characterization and structured integration of medical information to solve the problem of fragmentation of medical information data, through big data analysis and deep learning, accurate extraction and effective analysis of imaging graphic features that are easily ignored or difficult to distinguish by humans, so as to complete the prediction of lesion area identification, disease classification, and development degree. Through deep mining of massive digital information, extracting, refining, and quantifying individualized characteristics of diseases and parsing them, AI achieves a leap from data to knowledge and from knowledge to intelligence, complementing the strengths of the intervener's expertise to achieve more objective, accurate, and efficient clinical diagnosis and assessment.

As an important diagnostic basis that can accurately and intuitively reflect the apparent status of a condition, medical imaging, combined with the breakthroughs in deep learning technology in extracting image features, has become one of the areas where artificial intelligence is most closely integrated with assisted diagnosis. The accuracy of artificial intelligence diagnosis and analysis in Alzheimer's disease classification based on brain MRI, diabetic retinopathy detection based on fundus photographs, breast cancer lymph node metastasis detection based on digital pathological sections, skin cancer diagnosis based on skin photographs, and prognosis prediction based on tumor pathological features has reached or exceeded the level of professional doctors. In 2016, Gulshan team of University of California, USA reported for the first time in the journal *JAMA* that the use of artificial intelligence to diagnose diabetic retinopathy from more than 100,000 retinal fundus photographs has significantly improved the sensitivity and specificity compared to professional ophthalmologists. In 2018, Google DeepMind system can not only diagnose a single disease, but also identify 50 different eye diseases based on its analysis of imaging data. It can also analyze three-dimensional scanning imaging. Compared to the artificial intelligence system that can only identify two-dimensional images, it can process more data information. Cardio DL system is the first artificial intelligence diagnostic analysis system based on deep learning approved by FDA. This system performs deep learning for more than 1000 MRI images based on convolutional neural network algorithm, and summarizes ten million related patterns, which can more accurately identify cardiac lesions. Cardio DL may reduce the diagnostic speed from 30 min of professional physicians to 15 s. The ContaCT system is the first FDA-approved artificial intelligence diagnostic decision system for stroke. ContaCT summarizes the image pattern most closely related to stroke by learning the brain CT images of stroke patients. In clinical trials, the sensitivity and characteristics of ContaCT in identifying large vessel obstruction were 90%, and the time from CT image generation to physician obtaining reminder was less than 6 min, which gained time for successful treatment of patients. Cognoa is the first artificial intelligence diagnostic decision support system for children with autism. By analyzing the information and video of children's natural behavior provided by parents, Cognoa system can evaluate the children's mental and behavioral health status through artificial intelligence machine learning and improve the timeliness of children's autism diagnosis and treatment.

5.3.2 Influence on Pathological Diagnosis of Tumor

Pathological diagnosis is the gold standard for clinical treatment. However, traditional pathological diagnosis is not easy to quantify, has a great dependence on the experience of pathologists, and has a great impact on subjective factors in the diagnosis. The standardization and uniformity of pathological diagnosis have been unable to meet the needs of clinical development. At present, artificial intelligence pathology has made new breakthroughs in tumor cytology primary screening, benign and malignant differentiation, morphometric analysis, and histological classification, and can even achieve early diagnosis of cancer, precancerous lesions, and even latent tumors on imaging and blood data, creating conditions for early treatment. The Esteva team at Stanford University used 129,450 clinical images containing data from 2032 different skin diseases and performed migration learning based on Google TensorFlow using the Inception V3 model to achieve diagnostic accuracy of over 90% for both skin cancer and melanoma. The research results have been applied through smartphones and can effectively detect whether they have skin cancer, greatly saving the cost of medical testing. In 2018, nearly 150 scientists from more than 100 laboratories around the world jointly analyzed the methylation data of nearly 3000 tumor samples using artificial intelligence system in a study published in Nature and summarized the methylation characteristics of 82 central nervous systems, followed by traditional pathological analysis and artificial intelligence system analysis and comparison of 1104 samples. The results showed that 60.4% of the samples were completely consistent with the diagnosis, and 15.5% of the samples were basically consistent with the diagnosis. This study shows that artificial intelligence can improve the qualitative and quantitative judgment level of pathology and improve the accuracy of pathological diagnosis.

In addition to pathological diagnosis by feature extraction of pathological image data, artificial intelligence can also construct an intelligent prediction model combining multimodality data acquisition analysis with structured knowledge inference to individualize the prediction of disease development and patient prognosis. In 2016, Nature Communication reported a study of artificial intelligence to predict the prognosis of cancer patients. The study included digital images of 2186 tissue sections of lung adenocarcinoma and lung squamous cell carcinoma and images of 294 tissue microarray databases in the Cancer and Tumor Genetic Atlas (TCGA) database, first extracted 9879 quantitative features from pathological images, and then screened the top features by machine learning algorithms, which could well predict the survival time of patients with lung adenocarcinoma and lung squamous cell carcinoma.

In terms of molecular pathology, the traditional genetic detection methods have been unable to meet the needs of multiple genetic detection, and the emergence of new technologies such as high-throughput sequencing provides a new opportunity for the accurate treatment of tumors. Genetic testing by high-throughput sequencing can evaluate the prognosis of tumors with different gene mutations and determine the sensitivity of chemotherapy and targeted drug therapy, which has shown the superiority of artificial intelligence in the precise treatment of tumors such as breast cancer, lung cancer, and colon cancer. Therefore, the application of artificial intelligence technology to analyze massive genomics information has become an indispensable element in the development of cancer therapy.

5.3.3 Impact on Clinical Decision-Making Modes

In traditional clinical decision-making, the decision level of intervention providers mainly relies on the accumulation of personal experience as well as longitudinal and horizontal learning ability. To make correct and rapid clinical judgment and decision-making for complex and variable conditions, intervention providers need a lot of literature reading, following the frontiers of disciplines, long-term unremitting training and accumulation of clinical experience. By learning massive medical data and professional knowledge, simulating the thinking and diagnosis and treatment methods of intervention providers, and synthesizing natural language processing, cognitive technology, machine learning, and other technologies, artificial intelligence is expected to have the decision-making ability of intervention providers and provide efficient and accurate diagnostic results and personalized treatment plans in a short time. However, it is important to note that the studies to date have only compared intelligent decision-making with intervention provider decision-making compliance rates and have not further explored the advantages and disadvantages of intelligent decision-making versus intervention provider decision-making and how intelligent decision-making can be integrated with traditional clinical practice to bring clinical benefit to more patients. Therefore, in addition to exploring and improving the coincidence rate between artificial intelligence decision-making and intervention provider decision-making from the perspective of computer program and mechanical network principle, scientists need to further explore the impact of artificial intelligence decision-making system on different levels of hospitals and intervention providers and the possible impact on the clinical benefits of patients from the perspective of medical humanities and treatment, and include the intervention provider factors into the scope of consideration, so as to better apply artificial intelligence to clinical decision-making.

5.3.4 Remote and Intelligent Robotic Surgery System

Artificial intelligence surgical robots mainly include four major technologies: robotic technology, visualization technology, instruments, and data analysis. Da Vinci surgical robotic-assisted system developed by Intuitive Surgical, USA is currently a representative and most widely used surgical robotic system, which brings great technological changes to minimally invasive surgery. The 3D high-definition imaging system can give the operating field a real depth sense, facilitate the intraoperative identification of anatomical layers, distinguish subtle structures, facilitate the flexible and stable operating arm to facilitate the implementation of fine operations such as separation, suture, and knotting, and significantly improve the accuracy and safety of surgery. The technical advantages of Da Vinci surgical robot overcome the limitations of traditional laparoscopic techniques and can maximize the advantages of minimally invasive surgery, which has been widely used in urology, cardiovascular surgery, obstetrics and gynecology and abdominal surgery. The first minimally invasive surgical robot system "Micro Hand S" jointly developed by Tianjin University and Wego in China that can realize modular assembly has completed the preliminary clinical trial and entered the registration testing stage in March 2017.

Most of the current role of surgical robots is limited to providing assistance for intervention providers in surgical procedures, and it is also necessary to further reflect the great promotion of surgery by artificial intelligence. The application of artificial intelligence is expected to use virtual reality technology to simulate the surgery for the images collected by different imaging systems before surgery, and use augmented reality technology to render the reconstructed lesions, functional areas, and other virtual reality information into the intraoperative visual image during surgery, realizing intraoperative real-time display, so as to improve the accuracy of surgery. For example, the spinal surgery-assisted robot MazorX improved the accuracy of spinal implantation surgery to 98.3% by introducing preoperative analysis, intraoperative guidance, and real-time three-dimensional verification techniques. In 2016, the STAR surgical robot completed animal experiments on end-to-end suturing of porcine small intestine without human assistance by fluorescently marking the surgical position, becoming the world's first fully automated surgical robot. In June 2018, "Tianji", an orthopedic surgical robot with independent intellectual property rights in China, also completed the first orthopedic surgery. Through accurate positioning of the patient in three-dimensional space and intraoperative implementation of the virtual surgery plan to the specific patient, the surgical path is accurate, reducing the dependence on the experience of the intervention provider, improving the accuracy of the surgery and reducing the risk of difficult surgery.

In the future, artificial intelligence surgical robots will also realize independent learning function, convert different surgical video information into multimodal data through deep learning of a large number of surgical videos, and perform three-dimensional reconstruction of cloud images at lesion sites according to 3D visual information. The convolutional neural network will be used to repeatedly train a large number of three-dimensional point cloud images, so that the robots can automatically operate on the patients through the image feature matching and multisensor data fusion technology. Perhaps what the intervention providers need to do in the future is to control the surgical process and safety, further reducing the dependence on the experience and skills of the intervention providers and promoting the improvement of uneven allocation of medical resources.

5.4 Forecasts

At present, artificial intelligence is still in the era of weak artificial intelligence, and its application is in the field of image recognition-assisted diagnosis, which does not require man–machine communication. Using artificial intelligence to participate in the process of diagnosis and treatment, combining human intelligence with artificial intelligence and realizing expert empowerment of artificial intelligence is expected to transform artificial intelligence from a means of intervention to an intervention provider with decision-making and execution power, and build a new clinical intervention system with human–machine collaboration. Clinical intervention providers should be encouraged to become the participants, practitioners, and innovators of artificial intelligence medical treatment. Using human intelligent cognition to empower the knowledge system of artificial intelligence system, in turn, artificial intelligence can also improve the cognitive level of intervention providers to the medical field, improve the uncertainty of medical behavior and improve the prognosis of patients. Artificial intelligence technology should also be able to develop a set of standard treatment and decision-making system suitable for Chinese patients according to the disease characteristics of Chinese population, combined with clinical guidelines and evidence-based medical evidence, develop an authoritative individualized diagnosis and treatment plan for Chinese patients, and improve the differences in the uneven diagnosis and treatment level of medical institutions at all levels. The future artificial intelligence will bring profound changes to the medical field, change the medical technical means, and even the diagnosis and treatment model, and become a strong impetus for future medical innovation and development.

5.4.1 Intelligent Medical Image Recognition and Prediction

Intelligent medical image recognition aims to analyze and process commonly used medical images such as CT, MR, and surgical videos through deep neural networks and convolution learning techniques, with the purpose to improve the efficiency and quality of image recognition and then provide help for diagnosis and treatment.

At present, the recognition of intelligent medical images mainly focuses on organ recognition, vascular segmentation, pathological section analysis, pathological analysis based on medical images, surgical video content analysis, and other aspects. Among them, identifying the target region from the image is the first and core step of intelligent medical image processing. In order to achieve accurate target recognition, a variety of artificial intelligence methods have emerged, such as the method of training the machine through manual labeling followed by machine autonomous learning, or image recognition through the spatial relationship with adjacent large organs, or the use of iterative methods to identify the target area through rough segmentation and fine segmentation through two neural networks successively. These methods have their own advantages and disadvantages. Simple methods tend to have low recognition efficiency, while more complex methods have the disadvantages of excessive computation and high hardware requirements (Table 4.1).

The analysis of surgical video is another newly developed branch of intelligent surgery. Through the analysis of surgical video, the machine can understand the current surgical operation, so as to prompt the details of surgical operation and help the surgeon to make a reasonable choice for the next operation. Video analysis is a

Table 4.1 Differences between the three intelligent medical image recognition methods

Item	Machine learning model training	VOI (Volume of interest) method	Iterative method
Principle	After the manually labeled images are trained into machine learning models, the shapes and positions of organs are obtained, and then the organs are segmented near the positions	Firstly, the large organs adjacent to the small organs are located, and then the volume containing the target organs is determined according to the relationship between them, and then the segmentation operation is performed again	Using iterative method, coarse segmentation and fine segmentation are carried out successively through two neural networks
Pros	Simplified algorithm flow	Good identification of small organs	Good recognition rate for different organs
Cons	Poor recognition rate of small organs	Low recognition efficiency	Excessive operation, demanding hardware

manufacturing system that continuously collects and understands environmental information and its own information through self-learning function, continuously enriches the knowledge base in practice, and analyzes and judges its own behavior. In the future, surgical video analysis technology combined with 3D printing technology can assist in accelerating surgical learning of surgical medical students and shortening the training cycle of surgeons.

Due to the single way of medical data acquisition and the lack of training data and the difficulty to obtain it, there are still many problems in intelligent medical image recognition, such as narrow disease spectrum coverage and still need to improve the diagnostic accuracy. How to integrate resources, solve the problem of difficulty in obtaining medical data, and meet the large amount of data required by artificial intelligence is a critical problem in intelligent medical imaging research. At present, the author's team uses the two-step convolution neural network of vgg16 localization combined with inception identification to optimize the image postprocessing method, and further remove the false positive results through Z-axis continuity screening, which significantly improves the accuracy of pancreatic cystadenoma classification and diagnosis, and facilitates the selection of surgical decisions.

5.5 Three-Dimensional Reconstruction and Surgical Planning

Since the "Visible Human Project" was first proposed in the United States in the 1990s, three-dimensional virtual imaging technology has developed rapidly, and its application in the field of surgery has brought about a new surgical revolution. On the basis of high-precision CT and MR data, three-dimensional virtual imaging technology forms stereoscopic and complete organ and tissue images through digital three-dimensional reconstruction, which can truly reproduce the fine anatomical structure of organ and tissue and help doctors better understand, analyze the lesion and develop a surgical plan, so that the surgery can be performed more safely and effectively, reduce intraoperative risks and improve the prognosis of patients.

Three-dimensional reconstruction according to the plane data of the lesion site can truly reflect the location of the lesion and the anatomical relationship with blood vessels and organs. Through accurate observation and judgment of the lesions in the stereoscopic image data, it provides the doctor with decision support for the surgical plan. With the help of the surgical planning system, the preoperative evaluation is more accurate and the surgical plan is more scientific and individualized. At the same time, it helps doctors and patients to have more intuitive communication, and is of great significance to assist postoperative observation and effect evaluation.

In the future development, three-dimensional reconstruction technology will add more information, such as motion compensation, depth information, and compression perception, in order to be more in line with the actual situation. It can also be combined with MR (Mix Reality) technology and intraoperative navigation technology to project the three-dimensional reconstruction image of intraoperative surgical site in the surgical area in real time, so that it can be adjusted at any time with the change of real-time state of the patient as the surgical operation of the surgeon, so that the surgeon can more intuitively understand the anatomical structure of the surgical site and its real-time change, so that the surgical process is simpler and more direct, reducing the difficulty of surgery.

5.6 Intraoperative Navigation

Intraoperative navigation technology is a man–machine integrated intelligent system composed of intelligent machines and human experts. It uses computer, acoustic, radiological, optical, and electromagnetic technologies to provide intuitive images of surgical scenes including information such as key tissues or vascular positions fused by images through computer screens during physician surgery, so as to assist in the implementation of surgery. Intraoperative navigation is a new intersection of medicine and engineering technology and an ergonomically integrated hybrid intelligent system, which will expand, extend, and partially replace the mental work of human experts in the manufacturing process. Through intraoperative navigation, it can reduce the difficulty of surgery, improve the accuracy of surgery, reduce surgical complications, simplify complex surgery, and facilitate the development and promotion of some difficult surgeries. Surgical navigation systems were first applied in the field of neurosurgery, and later with the continuous development of navigation technology, their clinical scope has been gradually extended to spinal surgery, otorhinolaryngology, plastic surgery, etc., not only improving the quality of surgery but also making previously unfinished or high-risk surgery feasible.

Intraoperative navigation technology includes several key technologies: surgical planning systems, spatial localization techniques, and image registration. Planning systems allow for 3D surgical simulation in virtual space prior to surgery to develop a more complete surgical plan and allows for real-time comparison of surgical simulations during surgery. Spatial localization techniques can establish a close relationship between the patient, surgical scene, and preoperative images. Dynamic image registration is the most important step of intraoperative navigation. During the operation, the surgeon and the tissues and organs in the surgical target area are in the process of changing the relative position. Through dynamic registration, the machine continuously tracks and identifies the target of changing position.

In order to achieve anterior image fusion and accurate registration during surgery, different intraoperative navigation systems need to be selected. In the use of navigation system, the precision requirement shall be higher than 1.5 mm. The current navigation system is divided into three categories: optical navigation system, electromagnetic navigation system, and hybrid navigation system. The means of optical navigation system tracking is mainly through the reflection of infrared rays from the object, which has the advantages of higher tracking accuracy and longer acting distance, but it cannot work properly if it is blocked by other objects. Electromagnetic navigation systems do not have the limitation of optical system "occlusion" and can also be tracked in the human body, but the action distance is limited. The hybrid navigation system makes full use of the advantages of the above two and overcomes the disadvantages of the two as far as possible, but because of more equipment, it increases the complexity of the system, easily produces system errors, and is expensive. In the future development, intraoperative navigation will be continuously studied from several core technologies such as how to reduce the delay rate, improve accuracy, and improve modeling efficiency, solve the current situation that the development of intraoperative navigation technology does not match the needs of clinical practical application, and develop intraoperative navigation equipment with independent intellectual property rights in China.

5.7 Remote and Intelligent Robotic Surgery System

Robotic surgery system originated from remote surgery. In 2000, Intuitive Surgical successfully developed Da Vinci Surgical System with three-dimensional visualization and human–machine interface, which opened the attempt of robot in the field of surgery and provided a platform for remote and intelligent operation of surgery. At present, the development of computer, remote communication, Internet and surgical robot technology lays a foundation for the realization of remote surgery. On the one hand, remote robotic surgery can enable patients to receive the treatment of optimal surgeons as early as possible, which is conducive to grasping the best treatment timing and optimizing the allocation of medical resources; on the other hand, surgeons can continuously perform remote surgery for multiple patients located in different places, which is helpful to improve the treatment efficiency. However, remote surgery technology is still in the stage of animal experiments and clinical trials, and still faces a series of problems such as delayed information transmission, high cost of training robotic surgical assistants and instrument nurses, unified robotic surgical methods yet, and restricted indications.

Intelligence is the core and difficulty in the development of robotic surgery system. Surgical robots should not only be the implementation tools of fine surgery but also should actively identify the location of lesions, develop surgical plans, and automatically implement surgery under the supervision of surgeons by analyzing a large number of real-time data with high dimensions and using more and more advanced sensors to realize the "full robotization" of surgery. This liberates the surgeon from being the surgeon who performs the surgery to being a supervisor.

Aiming at the characteristics of robotic surgical system in the circuit, we empower the design of new generation surgical robots with expert experience, address the shortcomings of current robotic surgical system such as lack of force feedback and low intelligence, propose R&D requirements and validation with rich clinical experience, and participate in the construction of new intelligent robotic surgical platform. The world's first 5G network-based telerobotic surgery was completed. Using 5G transmission technology and domestic robotic surgery system, remote hepatectomy surgery was performed on experimental animals, verifying the feasibility of telerobotic surgery under 5G technical conditions.

Suggested Reading

Bruno B, Tristan C. Computer go: an AI oriented survey. Artif Intell. 2001;132(1):39–103.

Cao J, Chen YJ. Combined liver transection and portal vein ligation for two-step hepatectomy: several focal points. Chin J Pract Surg. 2014;34(8):713–6.

Chen GT, Liu ZM. Theory and practice of damage control surgery. J Surg Concepts Pract. 2005;10(2):197–8.

Chen SD, Ran QH, Chen YH, Liao XQ. Clinical application of damage control surgery in severe abdominal trauma. Chin J Bases Clin Gen Surg. 2017;24(4):496–7.

Cui YY, Liu YF, Wang XW. Problems and discussion in practical application of cost-effective analysis. Chin Health Econ. 2015;34(9):8–9.

Han Y, Huang L, Shi T, Liu YB, Xu ZY, Sui L, Yu P, Xia Y, Geng ZC, Mao EQ, Wang XY. Application of damage control concept in abdominal emergency and trauma (report of 120 cases attached). J Surg Concepts Pract. 2018;23(2):155–8.

Jiang ZF, Xu FR. Artificial intelligence in the eyes of oncologists. J Precis Med. 2018;33(1):9–13.

Liu R. Opportunities and challenges in intelligent surgery. Chin J Surg Oncol. 2017;10(6):327–30.

Liu R. Reasonable selection and evaluation of laparoscopic hepatectomy approach. Chin J Laparosc Surg. 2018a;11(3):129–31.

Liu R. Entering into a new era of intelligent medicine. Chin J Surg Oncol. 2018b;11(2):65–8.

Liu R. Transformation of doctors in the era of intelligent medicine. J Laparosc Surg. 2018c;23(1):1–3.

Liu R, Hu MG. Discussion on several problems of laparoscopic anatomical hepatectomy: 10-year experience of Chinese PLA general hospital. Chin J Surg. 2010;3(6):466–73.

Liu Q, Liu R. Intraoperative risk control and minimally invasive Hepatopancreatobiliary surgery. Chin J Laparosc Surg. 2017;10(2):65–8.

Liu R, Zhang X. Strategies and key points of laparoscopic surgery for severe acute pancreatitis. Chin J Pract Surg. 2015;35(5):493–5.

Liu R, Zhao GD. Liver anatomy: from the trunk theory under static anatomy of cadavers to the watershed theory under morphology of clinical potential. Chin J Laparosc Surg. 2018;11(05):257–60.

Liu R, Zhao GD, Ma X, Hu MG, Wang W. Application of retroperitoneoscopic technique in surgical treatment of severe acute pancreatitis. Chin J Laparosc Surg. 2010;3(4):309–12.

Liu YY, Lai JX, Liu XX. Changes in the concept of surgical treatment of liver cancer from the evolution of ALPPS. Chin J Pract Surg. 2016;36(6):593–5.

Liu R, Yin ZZ, Zhao GD. Transition of surgical intervention strategy for severe acute pancreatitis. J Laparosc Surg. 2017;8:561–3.

Liu R, Liu Q, Zhao ZM, Tan XL, Gao YX, Zhao GD, Xu Y, Yin ZZ. Application of single-needle full-layer pancreaticojejunostomy (301 type) in pancreaticoduodenectomy. J Laparosc Surg. 2018;23(11):853–7.

Mezger U, Jendrewski C. Bartels MJLsaos. Navig Surg. 2013;398(4):501–14.

Tian WH. Cost-benefit and cost-effective analysis. J Hosp Manag Chin People's Liber Army. 1995;2(1):76–9.

Wang F, Liu R. Intelligent surgery: changing trends in surgical practice patterns. Acad J Second Milit Med Univ. 2018;39(8):830–4.

Wang XF, Hu MG, Zhao GD, Xu Y, Xu DB, Xue RH, Liu R. Exploration of a laparoscopic standard: patterned laparoscopic left hemihepatectomy. Chin J Surg Oncol. 2014;7(3):160–6.

Wang HX, Tian XQ, You M, Lu XQ, Gu ZL, Cheng L. Application status, problems and suggestions of artificial intelligence in medical field. Soft Sci Health. 2018;32(5):3–7.

Xu N, Tian LY, Wang XY. Cost-benefit analysis of diagnosis and treatment of hypertension. Chin J Bone Joint Surg. 2017;10(6):496–8.

Yan LN. Current status and prospect of application of artificial intelligence in medical field. Chin J Bases Clin Gen Surg. 2018;25(5):513–4.

Yang WB, Meng QM. Application of cost-benefit analysis in hospital economic management. Econ Res Guid. 2018;16:110–1.

Yu GZ, Liu XY, Zhang YC, Yang JD, Tian JH, Zhu MH. Application and thinking of artificial intelligence in clinical medicine. Acad J Second Milit Med Univ. 2018;39(4):358–64.

Zhang ZH, Gao JZ. Significance and methods of implementing clinical paths. Chin J Hosp Admin. 2002;18(9):513–9.

Zhang WQ, Long X. Damage control and tumor-free operation strategy in hepatectomy for liver cancer. Chin J Pract Surg. 2018;38(4):367–73.

Zhao GD, Liu R. Teaching and practice of trocar arrangement method in robotic hepatopancreatobiliary surgery. Chin J Surg Oncol. 2018;11(3):166–71.

Zhao GD, Hu MG, Liu R. Patterned laparoscopic left lateral lobectomy: a report of 71 cases. J South Med Univ. 2011;4:737–40.

The Choice of Intervention Timing

5

Rong Liu and Qu Liu

Abstract

Timing of intervention is crucial, and different timings of intervention may lead to diametrically opposite outcomes. This chapter describes the relationship between disease risk, intervener, and interventions and the timing of intervention. The relationship between disease risk and intervention timing is to explain how to grasp the timing of intervention according to the disease risk through different stages of the development of the same disease. In the section of interveners and intervention timing, two examples are used to elaborate how interveners influence intervention timing. In the section of intervention means and intervention timing, two examples are also used to illustrate the importance of choosing intervention timing according to the fit of interveners and interventions.

1 Disease Risk and Intervention Timing

In the Introduction section, we introduce the concept, classification, and principles of the timing of intervention. In this section, we tell how to select the appropriate timing of intervention according to the risk of disease from the perspective of disease risk and through specific clinical cases. Disease risk is the intervention object of prognosis control medicine, and controlling disease risk is also the primary goal of prognosis control medicine. Therefore, the criticality and severity of disease risk determine the grasp of the timing of intervention. In the complex clinical work, the situation of admitting multiple patients at the same time is often encountered. The

R. Liu (✉) · Q. Liu
Faculty of Hepato-pancreato-biliary Surgery, Chinese PLA General Hospital, Beijing, China
e-mail: liurong301@130.com

R. Liu (ed.), *Clinical Decision Making for Improving Prognosis*,
https://doi.org/10.1007/978-981-19-2952-6_5

intervention provider must master the ability to accurately determine the risk of the disease and quickly determine the timing of the intervention and implement the intervention according to the priority of the disease, otherwise it will affect not only the normal progress of clinical work but also the intervention effect of patients. In this section, we explain how to grasp the timing of intervention according to the risk of the disease by the different periods of disease development.

1.1 Case 1

The patient, a 28-year-old man, was admitted to the hospital with multiple gallstones found by B-ultrasonography during physical examination. Physical examination: temperature 36.5 °C, pulse rate 65 bpm, respiratory rate 16 bpm, blood pressure 128/75 mmHg. He was clearly conscious, cooperative on physical examination, with normal development, acceptable nutritional status, and no yellowing of the skin and sclera. The abdomen was flat, the liver and spleen were not palpable under the ribs, no palpable mass, no tenderness in the whole abdomen, no rebound tenderness, bowel sounds were normal, and shifting dullness was negative. The blood, urine, and stool routine were all normal. Blood biochemistry showed total bilirubin 15 umol/L, direct bilirubin 8 μmol/L, alanine aminotransferase 30.5 U/L, aspartate aminotransferase 25.5 U/L, serum albumin 40 g/L, alkaline phosphatase 40 U/L, and γ-glutamyltransferase 35 U/L. Abdominal ultrasound revealed a gallstone measuring about 0.5 × 0.5 cm. The patient complained of no usual symptoms of abdominal pain, abdominal distension or dyspepsia. Combined with the patient's symptoms, physical examination, and auxiliary examination, multiple gallstones were diagnosed. The author often encounters such patients in the outpatient clinic and comes to the hospital immediately after physical examination reveals gallstones. Considering the young age of the patient, the current gallbladder stones do not bring discomfort to the patient, and the size of the gallbladder stones does not affect the normal function of the gallbladder, if surgical intervention is performed at this time, it might affect their quality of life in future, and the loss and risk caused by the intervention would be much greater than the benefit of the intervention for young people, so the author would usually advise the patient to have a light diet and regular review.

1.2 Case 2

The patient, a 45-year-old man, was admitted to the hospital with persistent tingling in the right upper quadrant of the abdomen associated with nausea and vomiting for 3 h. Physical examination: temperature 38.1 °C, pulse rate 88 bpm, respiratory rate 21 bpm, blood pressure 138/75 mmHg. He was clearly conscious, cooperative on physical examination, with normal development, forced posture, acceptable nutritional status, and no yellowing of the skin and sclera. The abdomen was flat, the liver and spleen were not palpable under the ribs, no palpable mass, tenderness and rebound tenderness in the right upper quadrant were evident, bowel sounds were normal, and shifting dullness was negative. The blood, urine, and stool routine were all normal. Blood biochemistry showed total bilirubin 18 umol/L, direct bilirubin 10 μmol/L, alanine aminotransferase 65 U/L, aspartate aminotransferase 50 U/L, serum albumin 39 g/L, alkaline phosphatase 55 U/L, and γ-glutamyltransferase 42 U/L. Abdominal ultrasound revealed significant gallbladder wall edema and multiple stones in the gallbladder, with the largest of about 1.2 cm. The patient complained of persistent stabbing pain in the right upper abdomen with nausea and vomiting after eating fatty foods, and the pain radiated to the right shoulder and could not be relieved by changing position, and similar symptoms had occurred several times before. Combined with the patient's symptoms, physical examination, and auxiliary examination, the patient was diagnosed with acute calculous cholecystitis. This patient is a typical case of cholecystolithiasis-induced acute cholecystitis, because cholecystolithiasis obstructs the cystic duct, resulting in bile retention in the gallbladder and secondary bacterial infection causing acute inflammation. When facing patients with definite stones and causing repeated clinical symptoms, the intervention provider needs to immediately decide to implement the intervention, give anti-infective symptomatic treatment and perform emergency laparoscopic cholecystectomy, because the implementation of emergency surgery is a reasonable clinical decision from the perspective of the intervention provider's clinical decision or evidence-based medical evidence. Since the patient has just had an attack for 3 h and the inflammation around the gallbladder is mild, the minimally invasive surgery performed at this time not only has relatively low surgical risk but also can completely solve the root cause of the disease through radical surgery, avoiding recurrent attacks of cholecystitis in the future and improving the quality of life of the patient. Of course, some patients will be relatively resistant to surgery and afraid of surgical treatment. At this time, it is necessary for intervention providers to explain the development of the disease, the advantages and disadvantages of various intervention means and the possible impact on patients after surgery in detail, eliminate the concerns of patients, and strive to solve the problem in time with minimally invasive means.

1.3 Case 3

The patient, a 42-year-old woman, was admitted to the hospital with a 7-day history of intermittent distension and pain in the right upper quadrant. Physical examination: temperature 37.2 °C, pulse rate 75 bpm, respiratory rate 18 bpm, blood pressure 130/70 mmHg. The patient had clear consciousness, cooperation, normal development, normal body position, good nutritional status, and no jaundice of skin or sclera. The abdomen was flat, the liver and spleen were not palpable under the ribs, no palpable mass, mild tenderness in the right upper quadrant, no rebound tenderness, bowel sounds were normal, and shifting dullness was negative. The blood, urine, and stool routine were all normal. Blood biochemistry showed total bilirubin 15 μmol/L, direct bilirubin 8 μmol/L, alanine aminotransferase 38 U/L, aspartate aminotransferase 30 U/L, serum albumin 37 g/L, alkaline phosphatase 45 U/L, and γ-glutamyltransferase 37 U/L. Abdominal ultrasound revealed significant edema of the gallbladder wall, unclear display of the surrounding tissue, and a gallbladder filled with stones, with the largest of about 0.8 cm. Combined with the patient's symptoms, physical examination and auxiliary examination, the patient was diagnosed with acute calculous cholecystitis. This patient has a similar disease to the previous patient, and the biggest difference is that the duration of the disease is different, and the pathophysiological characteristics of the lesion will change significantly within this 7-day period, and the risk of surgical intervention will increase exponentially, thus resulting in different timing of intervention. Because more than 48 h after the onset of acute cholecystitis, the gallbladder and surrounding tissues have severe inflammation and edema, which are easy to adhere to the surrounding tissues and organs. If the surgical intervention is reluctantly implemented, it is easy to cause serious complications such as intraoperative bile duct and vascular injury. Once these intraoperative complications occur, they are difficult to recover, which will further lead to a series of serious complications such as bile leakage, liver dysfunction, and even liver failure. The patient was given conservative treatment such as anti-inflammation and fluid infusion. After 3 months, the inflammatory edema of gallbladder and surrounding tissues was alleviated, and the risk of intervention was significantly reduced, minimally invasive surgery was performed. Currently, with the development of laparoscopic techniques and the accumulation of surgical experience of operators, there is a trend to perform laparoscopic cholecystectomy also in the inflammatory edema phase. The author is not opposed to attempts to broaden the indications for treatment in order to achieve patient benefit, but the premise needs to be based on a full understanding of the disease, full preparation for the intervention, and full exercise of one's own abilities, and only when the benefits that the intervener and the intervention can bring to the patient outweigh the possible risks of the intervention does it not violate the medical principles and can truly bring benefit to the patient.

1.4 Case 4

The patient, a 65-year-old man, was admitted to the hospital with a 1-day history of persistent distension and pain in the right upper quadrant with nausea and vomiting. Physical examination: temperature 39.6 °C, pulse rate 96 bpm, respiratory rate 22 bpm, blood pressure 150/95 mmHg. He was indifferent, uncooperative on physical examination, in a forced position, in an acceptable nutritional state, with slightly yellowish staining of the skin and sclera. The abdomen was distended, the liver and spleen were not palpable under the ribs, no palpable mass, tenderness and rebound tenderness in the right upper quadrant were evident, bowel sounds were active, and shifting dullness was negative. Blood routine showed white blood cell 21.2×10^9/L, neutrophil ratio 95%, blood biochemistry showed total bilirubin 65 μmol/L, direct bilirubin 50 μmol/L, alanine aminotransferase 365 U/L, aspartate aminotransferase 350 U/L, serum albumin 32/L, alkaline phosphatase 155 U/L, and γ-glutamyltransferase 242 U/L. Abdomen CT revealed marked edema of the gallbladder wall and multiple stones in the gallbladder, with the largest of about 0.5 cm. The common bile duct was dilated, edema was obvious, and multiple stones were found. The patient complained of multiple previous history of cholecystitis development, and developed persistent swelling pain in the right upper quadrant with nausea, vomiting, high fever, and chills after eating greasy food. The pain radiated to the right shoulder. The condition further worsened after 1 day of conservative treatment in another hospital. Combined with the patient's symptoms, physical examination, and auxiliary examination, the patient was diagnosed with (1) acute obstructive suppurative cholangitis and (2) acute calculous cholecystitis. This patient is a typical case of acute obstructive septic cholangitis induced by gallbladder stones, because the original gallbladder stones were not thoroughly treated, resulting in the formation of impaction after the stones were discharged into the common bile duct, thus causing high pressure in the bile duct and retrograde bacteria in the bile into the blood, which is more dangerous and can lead to infectious shock, systemic inflammatory response syndrome, multi-organ failure, and even death of the patient. This type of disease has a rapid onset and rapid development, and once the timing of intervention is delayed, it may cause extremely serious consequences, so intervention providers need to pay extreme attention, make rapid clinical decisions after weighing the advantages and disadvantages, and seize the fleeting timing of intervention to implement therapeutic intervention. The patient's condition was further aggravated after 1 day of conservative treatment in an outside hospital. According to the occurrence and development of the disease and a large number of clinical experience, if conservative treatment was continued, there may be a risk of rapid change of the condition leading to a variety of serious complications. Therefore, the author team performed emergency choledochotomy, cholecystectomy, and T-tube drainage for the patients, which rapidly reduced the patient's symptoms through surgical treatment and avoided the occurrence of risks. Only in the face of such emergency critical illness can the intervention provider's ability to grasp the timing of intervention be reflected, the intervention provider needs to pay attention to accumulating experience in dynamically identifying the risk of such diseases at ordinary times, and improve the ability to implement clinical intervention in emergencies, and most importantly, he/she also needs to be vigilant and alarm at all times, in order to accurately grasp the timing of intervention when the risk appears to achieve accurate intervention.

2 Interveners and Intervention Timing

The intervention provider is the main body of the whole medical process, which is not only the implementer of the intervention means but also the determinant of the timing of the intervention, and plays a leading role in the whole prognosis control medical system. How do intervention providers influence the timing of interventions through their own factors? Do different intervention providers choose the same timing of intervention for the same disease risk? Is the optimal timing of intervention also the same for the same intervention provider in different states, different scenarios? This section will elaborate through two examples how intervention providers have an impact on the timing of the intervention.

2.1 Case 1

The patient, a 68-year-old woman, was admitted to the hospital with abdominal distension and abdominal pain associated with fever for 12 h. Physical examination: temperature 39.0 °C, pulse rate 98 bpm, respiratory rate 20 bpm, blood pressure 145/95 mmHg. She was clearly conscious, cooperative on physical examination, with normal development, acceptable nutritional status, and normal body position. She had no yellowing of the skin and sclera. The abdomen was flat, the liver and spleen were not palpable under the ribs, no palpable mass, mild tenderness around the umbilicus, insignificant rebound tenderness, hyperactive bowel sounds, and negative shifting dullness. Blood routine showed white blood cells 20.1×10^9/L, neutrophil percentage 92%, and normal blood biochemistry and coagulation function. Gas levels were observed in standing abdominal radiographs, and local intestinal dilatation of the small intestine was observed on abdominal CT. The patient complained of appendectomy 20 years ago, with persistent abdominal distension and pain, without radiating pain, accompanied by fever, nausea, no vomiting, no defecation or exhaust, and normal urination. Combined with the patient's symptoms, physical examination, and auxiliary examination, the patient was diagnosed with (1) adhesive intestinal obstruction and (2) s/p appendicectomy. When the patient visited the emergency department, the doctor on duty found through conversation with the patient and physical examination that the patient was in good general condition, free movement and no passive position. Considering that the patient's adhesive intestinal obstruction was mild and did not require surgical intervention, the patient was recommended to stay in the hospital for observation, and given fasting, gastrointestinal decompression, fluid replacement, and other symptomatic and supportive treatment. One hour later, when the superior doctor performed ward round, it was found that the patient's abdominal symptoms and signs were not obvious, but the fever symptoms were obvious and white blood cells and neutrophils continued to be at a high level, so emergency exploratory laparotomy was immediately decided. During the operation, it was found that the patient had developed intraabdominal hernia, small intestinal canal impaction, and constrictive necrosis. After partial bowel resection and adhesiolysis, the patient recovered well. In this case, the clinical decisions and timing of surgical interventions made by different intervention providers in the face of the same patient and the same disease were very different. In the end, the superior physician predicted the risk of strangulated intestinal obstruction in advance, made timely decisions and intervened immediately to avoid serious complications such as intestinal necrosis and perforation, and saved the patient from the death line.

Intestinal obstruction is a common acute abdomen. For most intervention providers, the diagnosis of intestinal obstruction is not difficult, and the treatment principles are not difficult to master. However, in clinical practice, the most difficult thing is to grasp the timing of surgery, especially in the process of conservative treatment. When should surgery be performed and when can conservative treatment be applied? How to diagnose and treat intestinal necrosis early before it occurs is the difficulty and focus of intestinal obstruction treatment. For adhesive intestinal obstruction caused by previous operations, if surgical treatment is performed rashly, the operation itself will also cause adhesion, and the adhesion caused by repeated operations will also increase the chance of recurrence of obstruction. However, if we take a chance and do not want to take the risk of surgery, the delayed surgery may cause intestinal necrosis and perforation, which may lead to infectious shock and multi-organ failure and death in serious cases. Therefore, this common disease of intestinal obstruction must not be careless and the timing of intervention needs to be carefully considered and weighed. For this patient, the young doctor on duty judged the development degree of the disease according to the typical characteristics of constrictive intestinal obstruction in textbooks and gave corresponding symptomatic treatment, which did not violate the medical principles in terms of diagnostic basis and treatment plan. However, not all patients with strangulated intestinal obstruction could fully show the above typical symptoms and signs in clinical practice. The patient's age, physical fitness, and patient's tolerance of the disease will show different clinical symptoms, and a large number of clinical practices need to be accumulated for the judgment of the specific timing of intervention. The superior physician, on the other hand, has extensive clinical experience and his own unique clinical thinking in the diagnosis and management of strangulated intestinal obstruction, judging the need for immediate surgical intervention based solely on the elderly patient, the more severe systemic inflammatory response, and the obscure signs and symptoms, avoiding more serious complications, protecting the patient's life, and reducing the overall economic burden on the patient. For the same case, different intervention providers have different grasps of the timing of intervention, which reflects the understanding of pathophysiological principles of the occurrence and development of the disease by different intervention providers, reflects the experience of different intervention providers in observing the symptoms, signs, auxiliary examinations, and other details of patients, and reflects the ability of different intervention providers to use clinical thinking and intervention means to control the risk of the disease and the risk of intervention. The impact of the timing of interventions on the risk of interventions is huge, especially in high-risk, fast-changing critical illnesses. Therefore, the timing of intervention requires higher demands on the intervention provider and the need to keep up with the times to find the best time to intervene.

Next we will tell about the impact of the intervention provider's own factors on the timing of the intervention by describing a case with some generality in the clinic.

2.2 Case 2

Director Wang of the Cardiac Surgery Department had a steady personality, exquisite surgical experience and skills, and was especially good at fine vascular suture. One morning, a risky and difficult coronary artery bypass surgery needed to be completed; however, the night before the surgery, Director Wang's father had a brain hemorrhage and was admitted to the intensive care unit for rescue. In order to ensure the successful completion of the surgery, although Director Wang did not sleep overnight, he still went to the operating table under great physical and psychological pressure. This beating heart bypass required the rapid completion of fine vascular anastomosis, which was a great test for the surgeon's psychology and technology. However, Director Wang had been excessively consumed by the physical and mental suffering the night before, the intraoperative observation, strain, and operation ability had been significantly reduced, it was difficult to achieve concentration, and it was thrilling. There was no danger, and finally, with his long experience, solid basic skills, and tenacity, Director Wang successfully completed the surgery.

In this case, the situation of Director Wang is not a single case in clinical practice, and even there will be reports in the society that this spirit of giving up a small family for patients is widely praised. However, for patients and intervention providers, is it a correct intervention opportunity to insist on working with illness similarly? Once the intervention risk caused by the psychological and physical problems of the intervention provider threatens the life safety of the patient, is this spirit worthy of praise? From the perspective of prognosis control surgery, the intervention provider is dominant in the intervention, and the intervention provider's ability to intervene and grasp the timing of the intervention are essential for the control of disease risk. However, the attributes of intervention providers should not be ignored, and it should pay attention not only to their clinical decision-making and the optimization of intervention ability but also to the influence of their own state on intervention quality. People are emotional animals, which are easily disturbed by external and internal factors. Their emotional, psychological, and physiological states will directly affect the control of disease risks and the implementation of intervention measures. If the intervention is reluctantly implemented when the intervention provider's own state is not good, it will not only affect the effect of treatment but even threaten the life safety of patients. Therefore, when the intervention provider suffers from troubles similar to those encountered by Director Wang in this case, he can explain to the patient and his family, change the operation time, or replace the operator with the same ability, instead of reluctantly performing the operation, so as to control the intervention risk to the greatest extent, truly realize the benefit of the patient, and truly be responsible for the patient.

3 Interventions and Intervention Timing

Intervention is the specific implementation method of prognosis control surgery and the medium of action between intervention providers and patients. The optimization of intervention means is an important measure to improve the prognosis of patients. With the continuous update and development of intervention means, on the one hand, it can expand the "window period" of intervention timing and win more treatment opportunities for patients. However, on the other hand, advanced intervention means are also a double-edged sword. If it cannot be fully grasped by intervention providers, it may lead to the original reasonable intervention opportunity becoming out of date. Therefore, it is particularly important to choose a more reasonable intervention opportunity according to the fit of intervention providers and intervention means.

3.1 Case 1

A 52-year-old man was admitted to the hospital with recurrent cough for 8 years and progressive dyspnea for 3 years aggravated for 1 month. Physical examination: temperature 36.8 °C, pulse rate 90 bpm, respiratory rate 22 bpm, blood pressure 140/95 mmHg. He was bedridden, had significant dyspnea, severely limited physical activity, and had poor nutritional status. He had mild cyanosis of the lips and mouth, jugular venous anger, and low breath sounds. Wet rales were heard in both lower lungs, and Velcro rales could be heard. Arterial oxygen saturation was about 78% under oxygen inhalation with a binasal catheter. Lung CT showed interstitial fibrotic changes in the right lung, early interstitial fibrotic changes in the left lung, and infection in the lower part of both lungs. Blood gas analysis revealed a partial pressure of blood oxygen of 52 mm Hg. Echocardiography showed right cardiomegaly, pulmonary artery diameter 28 mm, pulmonary hypertension (80/35 mmHg), and left ventricular diastolic dysfunction. Combined with the patient's symptoms, physical examination, and auxiliary examinations, the patient was diagnosed with (1) respiratory failure, (2) idiopathic pulmonary fibrosis of right lung, and (3) infection in the lower part of both lungs. After consultation and discussion by respiratory and thoracic surgery experts, it is considered that both drugs and ventilators can no longer correct respiratory failure caused by idiopathic pulmonary interstitial fibrosis, and lung transplantation is urgently needed. While awaiting lung transplantation, extracorporeal membrane oxygenation (ECMO) bypass was performed via the femoral artery-femoral vein. After 226 h of ECMO bypass, the patient underwent lung transplantation, and right lung transplantation was successfully performed after 7 h of continued ECMO maintenance during the operation. After operation, the patient was successfully weaned from the ventilator and discharged with good recovery after symptomatic treatment with anti-infection, anti-rejection, and glucocorticoid.

This is a typical case in which the patient has access to treatment and regains new life through the advancement and optimization of intervention means. As a patient with idiopathic pulmonary fibrosis, this patient has developed respiratory failure that is also difficult to correct by ventilator during the long-term course of the disease. At this time, lung transplantation is the only treatment to save the patient. However, due to the serious shortage of donors, many patients may die due to lung infection, pulmonary hypertension, right heart failure, and other conditions while waiting for lung transplantation. The "window period" of intervention timing is very short, and most patients cannot obtain the chance of lung transplantation at all. With the progress of medical science and technology bringing about the upgrading of intervention means, ECMO, as a new extracorporeal circulation technology, oxygenates the blood in the body through artificial cardiopulmonary bypass, that is, membrane lung, and then returns the blood to the patient to play a role in cardiopulmonary function replacement and maintain the blood supply of human organ tissues. As an effective means of cardiopulmonary support, ECMO can maintain the heart and lung function of patients, improve tissue oxygen supply, prolong the time for patients with end-stage pulmonary disease to wait for lung transplantation, so that they can seize the chance of lung transplantation surgery and bring hope for patients to survive. Advanced intervention means can change the current treatment model, prolong the "window period" of timing of intervention, and gain time to wait and access to treatment for patients who otherwise require immediate intervention. Therefore, the best intervention time is relative rather than absolute. Intervention providers need to keep up with the forefront of medical development, give full play to the advantages of intervention means optimization, so that the time for intervention can be extended continuously, and strive for more ample, sufficient, and flexible intervention time for patients, so that more patients can enjoy the advantages of diagnosis and treatment and benefit of prognosis brought about by the reform of intervention means.

Next we will tell about the important impact of the intervention provider's mastery of different interventions on the timing of the intervention by describing a case that is somewhat representative in the clinic.

3.2 Case 2

Director Zhang of Liver Surgery Department was a well-known expert in China, with fast operation speed and less blood loss, which enjoyed high reputation in the industry and among patients and their families. One day, a patient with liver cancer came here and asked Director Zhang to perform laparoscopic liver cancer surgery for himself. However, it was indeed difficult for Director Zhang, because although laparoscopic liver resection is the development trend of liver surgery at present, Director Zhang was good at open liver resection, and he had only a few experiences in laparoscopic liver resection, and had not yet completed the learning curve of liver resection. It was indeed a test for Director Zhang to complete this difficult case of right posterior lobe tumor resection by laparoscopy. Faced with the trust of the patient and his family, Director Zhang could not refuse and performed laparoscopic hepatectomy for the patient. During the operation, due to the difficulty in exposing the right posterior lobe tumor and the difficulty in controlling the right hepatic venous bleeding during the operation, the patient was finally converted to laparotomy for resection of the right posterior lobe tumor of the liver.

In this case, the intervention provider is a suitable intervener with rich experience and exquisite skills in hepatectomy, and the chosen intervention means is laparoscopic surgery with less trauma to the patient at present, which should have been the best intervention combination and should have achieved ideal intervention results, but the final intervention results are not as satisfactory as planned, and the reason is that there is a problem with the cooperation between the intervention providers and intervention means, which leads to the inappropriate intervention timing. The issue that the best intervention provider is not good at the best intervention has never been considered by scholars before, especially since evidence-based medicine focuses more on the selection of the best intervention and the timing of the intervention, but the influence of the interventionist factor has not been fully considered. For Director Zhang, if laparotomy is selected at this time, it is undoubtedly the best time for intervention, but laparoscopic surgery is still in the learning period, and it is still difficult to complete this difficult operation of right posterior lobectomy. At this time, it is obviously not the best time for intervention to combine the intervention provider and intervention means reluctantly. If Director Zhang comes to implement this type of surgery after passing the learning curve, it may be possible for patients to obtain similar or better therapeutic effect as laparotomy. Therefore, in prognosis control surgery, the intervention provider, intervention means, and intervention timing are not all mechanically combined according to each optimal choice to obtain the best prognostic effect, but should organically select the most reasonable intervention timing and optimal configuration combination according to the cooperation and mastery proficiency between the intervention provider and intervention means and the ability of the intervention provider to navigate the intervention means.

Suggested Reading

Fu JZ, Zhang LJ, Yu ZL. Relationship between operation time and prognosis of acute severe cholangitis. J Capital Med Univ. 2007;28(1):14–6.

Hoopes CW, Kukreja J, Golden J, et al. Extracorporeal membrane oxygenation as a bridge to pulmonary transplantation. J Thorac Cardiovasc Surg. 2013;145(3):862–7.

Huang ZQ. Strive to improve the therapeutic effect on severe acute cholangitis. J Pract Surg. 1986;6:12.

Lafarge M, Mordant P, Thabut G, et al. Experience of extracorporeal membrane oxygenation as a bridge to lung transplantation in France. J Heart Lung Transplant. 2013;32(9):905–13.

Li JS. Improving the quality of adhesive small bowel obstruction surgery. Chin J Pract Surg. 2000;(8):4–6.

Li N. Emphasis on non-surgical treatment of intestinal obstruction after abdominal surgery. Chin J Pract Surg. 2008;(9):689–91.

Mao WJ, Chen JY. Application of extracorporeal membrane oxygenation in pretransplant support transition. Chin J Organ Transplant. 2011;2(4):209–16.

Schwenter F, Dominguez S, Meier R, et al. Acute small bowel obstruction: conservative or surgical treatment? Rev Med Suisse. 2011;7(300):1341–4, 1346–1347

Shi LP, Huang SH, Zheng ZH, Liu JR, Su YB. Timing analysis of operation for acute severe cholecystitis. Chin J Gen Surg. 2018;27(2):225–30.

Sun LN, Wang NF. Progress in clinical application of extracorporeal membrane oxygenation. Adv Cardiovasc Dis. 2013;34(3):416–9.

Wang K. Application progress of extracorporeal membrane oxygenation in lung transplantation. Pract J Organ Transplant. 2016;4(3):190–2.

Wu XT, Zhou Y. Timing of surgical treatment of intestinal obstruction. Chin J Pract Surg. 2008;28(9):695–6.

Zhang ZM, Wei WP, Liu Z, et al. Timing of laparoscopic surgery for acute calculous cholecystitis in the elderly. Chin J Oper Proced Gen Surg. 2016;10(5):406–9.

Strategies of Clinical Decision Making for Improving Prognosis

6

Rong Liu and Qu Liu

Abstract

In this chapter, four core strategies of prognosis control surgery are described in detail: bleeding control, surgical approach selection, resection techniques, and reconstruction techniques. In the bleeding control part, taking liver resection as an example, the pre-control of liver blood flow to reveal and control the blood vessels in the area to be resected was proposed, and the traditional concept of "mainly preventing bleeding" was replaced by "mainly hemostasis during operation." In the section of surgical approach selection, taking minimally invasive pancreatic surgery as an example, the importance of reasonable surgical approach selection to reduce surgical trauma was presented. In the resection techniques section, we describe how to achieve radical resection of the tumor in terms of integrity and operability. In the reconstruction techniques section, the optimization of two techniques, pancreatic-intestinal anastomosis and pancreatic duct repair, is used as examples to demonstrate how to optimize reconstruction techniques to accelerate the healing of each anastomosis, promote the recovery of organ function, reduce the incidence of postoperative complications, and also simplify the operation steps and shorten the operation time.

1 Bleeding Control Technology

Due to the criss-cross vascular distribution around the tissues and organs, as long as it is surgery, it will face the problem of bleeding. Whether it is simple body surface mass resection or complex pancreaticoduodenal surgery, if the bleeding cannot be well controlled, it will not only contaminate the surgical field and affect the surgical

R. Liu (✉) · Q. Liu
Faculty of Hepato-pancreato-biliary Surgery, Chinese PLA General Hospital, Beijing, China
e-mail: liurong301@131.com

R. Liu (ed.), *Clinical Decision Making for Improving Prognosis*,
https://doi.org/10.1007/978-981-19-2952-6_6

operation of the surgeon but also affect the postoperative recovery of patients. For cancer patients, intraoperative blood transfusion is even significantly associated with tumor recurrence. Therefore, controlling bleeding has been an eternal theme and core technology link in surgery. With the development of science and technology, surgery has entered the era of "energy surgery" from the era of "cold weapon." Advanced surgical instruments make bleeding control more calm and the surgical area clearer. However, bleeding control cannot rely solely on surgical instruments, but requires improved bleeding control techniques and optimized interventions under the guidance of the theory of prognosis control surgery, and the implementation of effective bleeding control is a key factor in determining the success or failure of surgery as well as patient prognosis. With the development of minimally invasive surgical techniques and equipment, minimally invasive surgery has become a routine in some surgical fields due to its characteristics of small injury and rapid recovery. Due to the magnifying effect of minimally invasive lens, once large intraoperative bleeding occurs, it will not only contaminate the surgical area, making the normal anatomical level difficult to distinguish and increasing the difficulty of surgery, but also more easily hit the confidence of the surgeon, greatly testing the psychology and emotion of the surgeon. Therefore, intraoperative bleeding is the main factor leading to conversion of minimally invasive surgery to laparotomy and postoperative complications, and minimally invasive surgery emphasizes the control of intraoperative bleeding.

Since the liver has two sets of hepatic blood inflow system and one set of hepatic blood outflow system, it is easy to cause intraoperative bleeding that is difficult to control, and the liver was once considered to be a forbidden area for surgery. With the understanding of hepatic vascular anatomy and the continuous development of bleeding control technology, hepatic blood flow occlusion has developed from the initial Pringle method of total hepatic blood flow occlusion to hemihepatic blood flow occlusion, hepatic blood outflow occlusion, subhepatic vein occlusion, and other methods. However, under minimally invasive surgical conditions, the limited operating space, the bottom-up tubular view, the diminished tactile information, and the leverage effect of the operation make intraoperative bleeding control very difficult and the progress of minimally invasive liver resection becomes difficult. In the practice of massive laparotomy and minimally invasive liver surgery, according to the law of hepatic vascularity and the characteristics of minimally invasive surgery, the author proposed the theory of prognosis control of hepatic blood flow in the area to be removed by exposure and control in advance and replaced the traditional concept of "intraoperative hemostasis" with "bleeding prevention."

The theory of hepatic blood flow prognosis control advocates the flexible use of open vascular occlusion technique to achieve prognosis control of blood flow in the region of the liver to be removed. The main steps are: (1) Combine with preoperative image data, determine the location of the lesion, the area to be removed by the liver, and the distribution of peripheral blood vessels, and develop a reasonable bleeding control plan in advance. (2) In the treatment of hepatic blood flow, the supplied hepatic pedicle is freed in advance according to the extent of the liver tissue to be removed to block, which can not only control the bleeding of the liver section during hepatectomy in advance but also prevent iatrogenic dissemination of the tumor. (3) Because anatomical variations of the hepatic artery and portal vein are not uncommon, in order to avoid damage to the vessels and bile ducts due to anatomical variations, the author recommends intrathecal anatomy. However, the method of intrathecal dissection requires the surgeon's surgical experience and skills, and if the anatomy of the hilum is not familiar, it will cause damage to the hilar duct. Therefore, extrathecal dissection or "bundle" dissection with a linear cutter stapler can be performed in cases of difficult hilar anatomy due to cirrhosis or tumor compression. (4) For the phenomenon that the ischemic line is inconsistent with Couinaud segment after regional hepatic pedicle occlusion, the author proposes a watershed theory that is more in line with the anatomical characteristics of hepatic blood flow, which believes that the target liver segment is supplied by the surrounding hepatic pedicle together and has a relationship between each other. Therefore, in the process of hepatectomy, the author recommends adjuvant first hepatic portal occlusion, by blocking the supply of adjacent liver and traffic branches to the target liver segment, so as to effectively control intraoperative bleeding. (5) For the occlusion of hepatic vein, the surgeon must choose according to the surgical needs and his/her own experience, does not reluctantly perform extrahepatic separation, can expose the root of hepatic vein during hepatectomy and then divide it together with a little liver parenchyma, which can reduce the risk of bleeding and gas embolism caused by hepatic vein tear.

Effective blood flow control can realize the bloodless state of the liver segment to be resected, maintain the normal blood flow supply of the remaining liver, avoid accelerating the liver transection rate in order to shorten the hilar blocking time, make the process of hepatectomy more convenient, implement fine anatomy, effectively reduce the trauma of surgery to patients, reduce the incidence of postoperative complications, and also facilitate the promotion and application of minimally invasive hepatectomy.

1.1 Case 1

A 55-year-old male patient was admitted due to intermittent swelling pain in right upper quadrant for more than 1 month. Physical examination: temperature 36.9 °C, pulse rate 68 bpm, respiratory rate 18 bpm, blood pressure 135/80 mmHg. He was clearly conscious, cooperative on physical examination, with normal development, acceptable nutritional status, and no yellowing of the skin and sclera. The abdomen was slightly distended, the liver and spleen were not palpable under the ribs, no palpable mass, mild tenderness in the right upper abdomen, no rebound tenderness, normal bowel sounds, and negative shifting dullness. The blood, urine, and stool routine were all normal. Blood biochemistry showed total bilirubin 25 μmol/L, direct bilirubin 15 μmol/L, alanine aminotransferase 38.5 U/L, aspartate aminotransferase 35.6 U/L, serum albumin 38 g/L, alkaline phosphatase 45 U/L, γ-glutamyltransferase 35 U/L, hepatitis B surface antigen, hepatitis B e antigen, and hepatitis B core antibody were positive, and tumor marker AFP

780 μg/L. Contrast-enhanced MRI of the abdomen revealed a mass in the right liver, about 8 × 10 cm, which was considered to be a malignant tumor in the right liver. The patient complained of a history of hepatitis B for 10 years without regular antiviral therapy. Combined with the patient's symptoms, physical examination, previous history of hepatitis B, AFP, and imaging examination, the patient was clinically suspected to have (1) hepatocellular carcinoma of the right liver; (2) viral hepatitis B. Through the assessment of the patient's general condition and systemic organ function, the patient had normal cardiopulmonary function, EOCG score was 0, and normal activity was not affected by the disease. Through the analysis of imaging data, the patient's tumor was mainly located in the right liver, no suspicious extrahepatic metastases were found, the liver function was Child A, and the patient could tolerate surgical treatment. The advantages and disadvantages of laparotomy and laparoscopic surgery were explained in detail to the patient and his family, and laparoscopic right hemihepatectomy was finally selected.

Before surgery, through three-dimensional image reconstruction, the author more clearly observed the branches and shape of hepatic vessels, understood the adjacent relationship between tumors and vessels and could calculate the remaining liver volume through virtual hepatectomy, and planned an efficient and accurate surgical resection plane in advance. During the operation, the right hepatohepatic pedicle was first freed by intrathecal anatomy, and the right hepatic artery and right hepatic portal vein were ligated and transected, respectively, to control the bleeding of the main feeding hepatic pedicle in advance. In the process of hepatectomy, auxiliary first hepatic portal occlusion was implemented to block the supply of adjacent liver and traffic branches to the liver and more effectively control section bleeding. The author freed the branches of segments 4 and 5 of the encountered hepatic vein along the section, determined the main hepatic vein at the confluence point of the branches, and then divided the hepatic parenchyma along the plane of the main hepatic vein course, which was easier to observe and judge the branches and course of the hepatic vein under the magnifying effect of the laparoscopic lens, and finally exposed the root of the right hepatic vein and then divided it together with a little hepatic parenchyma. The hepatic artery, portal vein, hepatic vein, and bile duct branches can be completely exposed by comprehensive application of hepatic blood flow blocking technique and energy device represented by harmonic scalpel and Biclamp. The smaller hemorrhage can be coagulated by energy device, and the larger hemorrhage can be ligated or clamped, respectively, so as to truly achieve exact hemostasis and fine operation.

With the gradual application of robotic surgery system, its high-definition 3D lens, flexible and stable operating arm, and reduced requirements for assistant cooperation make the learning curve of surgery significantly shortened, and even surgeons without laparoscopic surgery experience can master the skills of right hemihepatectomy. Therefore, intervention providers need to keep pace with the times, continuously learn and master new intervention means, update the intervention concept so as to realize the continuous optimization of patient prognosis.

2 Surgical Approach Selection

At the beginning of surgery, surgeons first face the problem of where this surgery should start, which involves the surgical approach. The surgical approach does not simply refer to the choice of route for performing the operation, but includes a series of surgical strategy planning including channel, route, and target exposure. The correct surgical approach can not only expose a better surgical field, reduce iatrogenic side injuries and complications, making the operation more successful, but also simplify the surgical operation and shorten the learning curve of the operation, facilitating the implementation and promotion of the operation.

In the selection of surgical approach, it is more representative to select the approach for pancreatic surgery, because the pancreas is located behind the abdominal organs, the location is deep, and there are many adjacent organs and blood vessels. When pancreatic surgery is performed, it is usually necessary to perform a wide range of anatomy and mobilization of the tissue structure around the pancreas, often accompanied by different degrees of collateral injury in this process. Therefore, pancreatic surgery is not only difficult to perform, but also has a higher incidence of serious postoperative complications than other surgeries. According to the different locations of pancreatic lesions and the characteristics of minimally invasive surgery, the author's team established an individualized minimally invasive pancreatic surgery approach system, including:

1. Pancreatic surgery via a retroperitoneal approach (Fig. 6.1): In the long-term treatment of severe acute pancreatitis, the author finds that even if the pancreas and surrounding necrotic tissue are cleaned again, the incidence of postoperative infection and multiple organ failure is not significantly improved, and secondary infection of pancreatitis and multiple organ failure are the greatest risks that

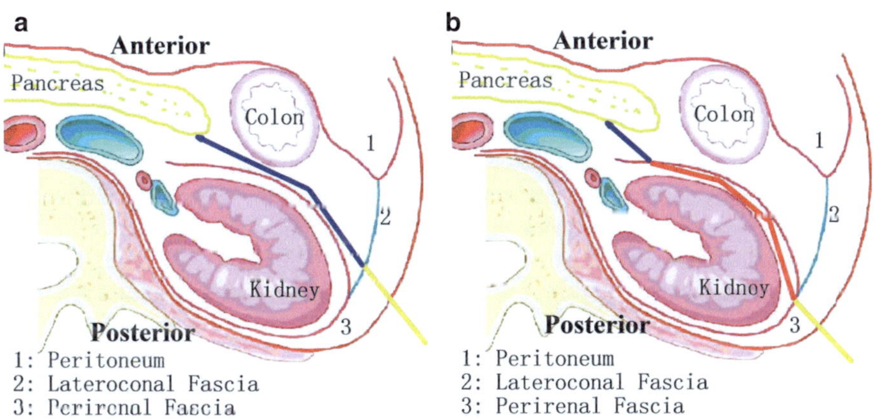

Fig. 6.1 Pancreatic surgery via retroperitoneal approach. (**a**) Side approach (through the posterior pararenal space, directly into the anterior pararenal space); (**b**) Posterior approach (through the posterior pararenal space, perirenal space, and finally into the anterior pararenal space)

severe pancreatitis surgery needed to face. How can this risk be pre-controlled within a controlled range? The author finds that the retroperitoneal space was limited and lacked the environment to activate trypsin. By referring to the retroperitoneoscopic resection of adrenal gland in urology, it could avoid entering the abdominal cavity, reduce the interference with the anatomical structure of normal peritoneal cavity, avoid the spread of abdominal infection, and the drainage path through the lateral posterior abdominal wall is direct and unobstructed, facilitating thorough and effective drainage. The author's team first introduced retroperitoneoscopic technique into pancreatic surgery, reducing the target injury and path injury of surgical intervention to patients, with high tolerance. With the innovation of its treatment concept, it has played a huge role in promoting the treatment of severe pancreatitis and significantly reducing the mortality of severe pancreatitis. Between the great advantages of retroperitoneoscopic approach in the treatment of severe pancreatitis, it can directly and rapidly expose the tail of the pancreas, and the author further applied it to the resection of tumors on the dorsal side of the tail of the pancreas. Because it is difficult for the traditional laparoscopic method to expose the lesions deep in the parenchyma of the tail of the pancreatic body, it is not only necessary to open the gastrocolic ligament, but also sometimes to transect the splenocolic ligament and the spleen and stomach ligament to expose the lesions. It is not only necessary to free and cut the original normal ligaments and fascial structures in the abdominal cavity, but also easy to cause damage to the middle colonic artery, colon, and splenic vein. The retroperitoneoscopic approach can avoid the above procedures and risks in advance, with the help of the pararenal space and perirenal space, directly reach the dorsal side of the pancreas, incise the anterior renal fascia behind it, and enter the anterior pararenal space from behind the space to expose the dorsal side of the caudal side of the pancreas. For prognosis control surgery, the most important thing is to find the shortest way to reduce the damage and interference to normal tissues. Selecting the correct surgical approach can not only avoid important tissues such as blood vessels and nerves, reduce the infestation and collateral injury to normal physiological structures, but also strengthen the control ability of intraoperative risks and avoid or reduce the occurrence of intraoperative and postoperative complications, which is conducive to the rapid recovery of patients.

2. Pancreatic surgery via the lesser omental bursa approach: When the tumor is located above the neck and body of the pancreas, the conventional surgical approach requires incision of the gastrocolic ligament to reach the neck and body of the pancreas. Due to the long path of this approach, more normal tissues need to be incised during surgery, especially when the greater omentum is hypertrophic or adherent, omental vascular bleeding is likely to occur during dissection, and even conversion to laparotomy due to injury to the transverse colon may occur, increasing the risk of surgery. The author can more quickly and safely expose the tumor located in the neck and body of the pancreas by using the lesser omentum approach, which can not only simplify the surgical procedures, but also avoid excessive tissue and vascular injury caused by the separation of the greater omentum, reduce the risk of intraoperative injury in patients, and accelerate the postoperative recovery of patients (Fig. 6.2).

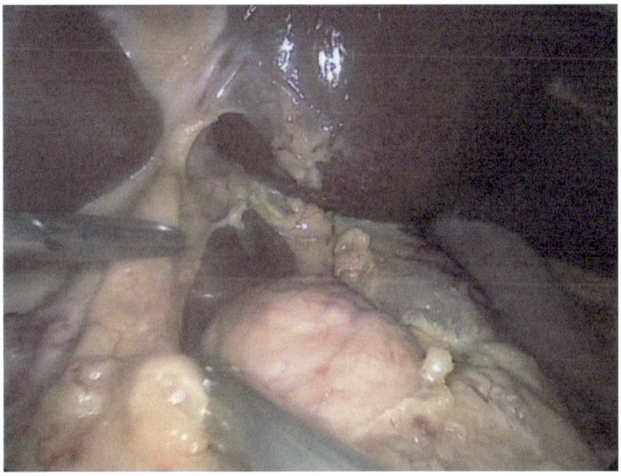

Fig. 6.2 Exposure of pancreatic body tumor via lesser omental bursa

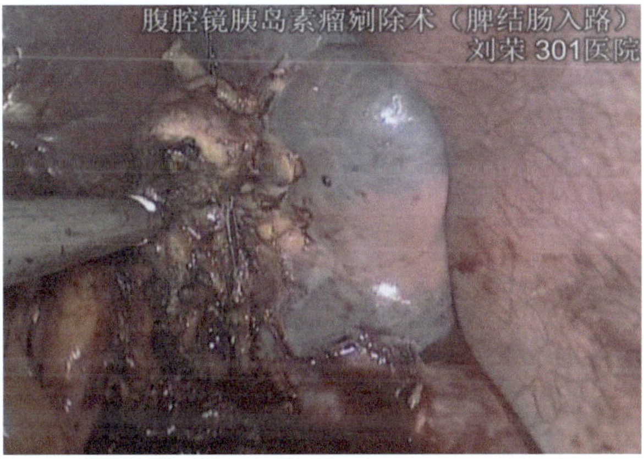

Fig. 6.3 Transsplenocolic ligament approach for resection of pancreatic tail tumor

3. Pancreatic surgery via the splenocolic ligament approach: For tumors located in the tail of the pancreas, the traditional surgical approach also has the above problems of large free range and more tissues involved, which easily leads to an increased incidence of postoperative complications and affects the prognosis of patients. The author directly dissociated the splenic colonic ligament through a trans-splenic colonic ligament approach, which can rapidly and safely reveal the caudal pancreatic lesion compared with the traditional approach (Fig. 6.3), effectively reduce the difficulty of minimally invasive surgery for caudal pancreatic tumors, accelerate the surgical process, and effectively reduce the incidence of intraoperative bleeding and postoperative complications.
4. Minimally invasive pancreaticoduodenectomy via L and R holes: However, under the condition of minimally invasive surgery, the lens vision and abdominal cavity space are limited, and it is difficult to invert the transverse colon, especially when the patient has thick transverse colon or more omental fat, it will lead to greater anastomosis tension and significantly increased operation diffi-

culty. Because the uncinate process of the pancreas is surrounded by the duodenum and its surrounding blood vessels are abundant, it is easy to block the surgical process due to bleeding during surgery. The treatment of the uncinate process of the pancreas is the focus and difficulty in pancreaticoduodenectomy. It is necessary to fully expose the uncinate process of the pancreas during surgery in order to reduce the risk of bleeding and ensure the positive rate of the resection margin. However, under the conditions of minimally invasive surgery, the space of surgical operation is limited, the range of motion of the device is small, and the surgical field is limited. According to the characteristics of these minimally invasive surgeries, the author's team has continuously explored and proposed the optimal approach to simplify the operation and improve the resection rate: the approach of the L-hole and R-hole (Fig. 6.4). L-hole approach: The L-hole is created by opening the transverse mesocolon on the left side of the superior mesenteric vessel, below the transverse colon, and on the left side of the middle colonic vessel. Through L-hole, without turning the transverse colon, the proximal empty field can be lifted to the posterior wall of the stomach for gastrointestinal anastomosis. It is the shortest path of gastrointestinal anastomosis, with small anastomotic tension and simple operation. It has become a routine approach for minimally invasive gastrointestinal anastomosis by the author's team. R-hole approach: The transverse mesocolon is opened from below the transverse colon, to the right of the middle colonic vessels, to establish the R-hole. Through this hole, the uncinate process of the pancreas and the descending and horizontal segments of the duodenum can be directly exposed, which reduces the difficulty of anatomical mobilization of the uncinate process of the pancreas and facilitates the local enucleation of the uncinate process tumor. By establishing an individualized minimally invasive pancreatic surgical approach, the advantages of minimally invasive surgery are utilized to reduce the risk of medically induced injury, decrease the incidence of postoperative complications,

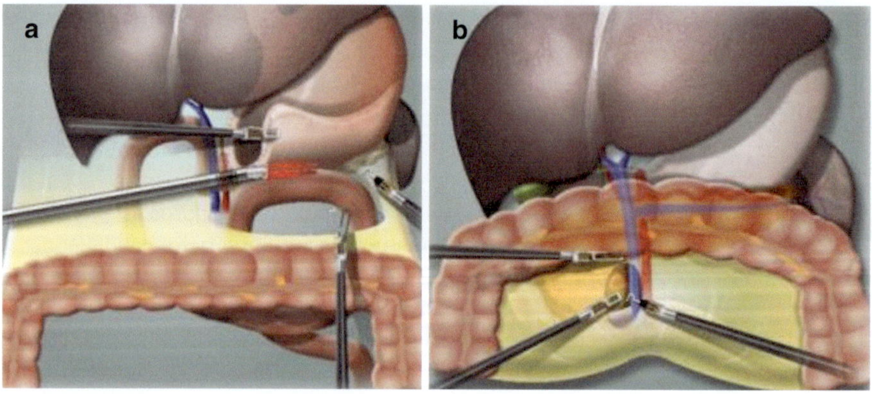

Fig. 6.4 Pancreatic surgery via L and R holes. (**a**) Gastrointestinal anastomosis via L-hole approach; (**b**) Exposed uncinate process of pancreas via R-hole approach

simplify the surgical operation method, and facilitate the rapid recovery of patients, and also facilitate the promotion and application of minimally invasive pancreatic surgery.

2.1 Case 1

A 26-year-old patient was admitted to the hospital with sudden onset of persistent abdominal pain after alcohol abuse. He had been treated conservatively at a local hospital for 2 weeks before admission and was transferred to our hospital with poor results. Physical examination: temperature 39.2 °C, pulse rate 85 bpm, respiratory rate 22 bpm, blood pressure 130/80 mmHg. He was clearly conscious, cooperative on physical examination, with normal development, acceptable nutritional status, and no yellowing of the skin and sclera. The abdomen was slightly distended, the liver and spleen were not palpable under the ribs, no palpable mass, mild tenderness in the middle and upper abdomen, with rebound tenderness, abdominal muscle tension, weak bowel sounds, and negative shifting dullness. Auxiliary examination showed white blood cells 14 × 109/L, neutrophil percentage 85%, urine amylase 860 U/dL, serum amylase 1500 U/dL, and serum lipase 850 U/L. Abdominal CT examination (Fig. 6.5) showed extensive necrosis of the pancreas (>50%), a large amount of retroperitoneal effusion, combined with pleural effusion and partial atelectasis. Combined with the patient's symptoms, signs, and auxiliary examination results, the patient was clinically diagnosed with severe acute pancreatitis. In this case, the patient with severe acute pancreatitis had a large amount of abdominal effusion and severe pancreatic necrosis, which had been operated and required removal of intra-abdominal necrotic tissue and unobstructed drainage. However, open surgery can cause the spread of infection while removing the pancreas and surrounding necrotic tissues, which can bring a second blow to the patient and even lead to multi-organ failure, and the mortality rate of acute severe pancreatitis has remained high. By investigating the causes and risks of postoperative deterioration

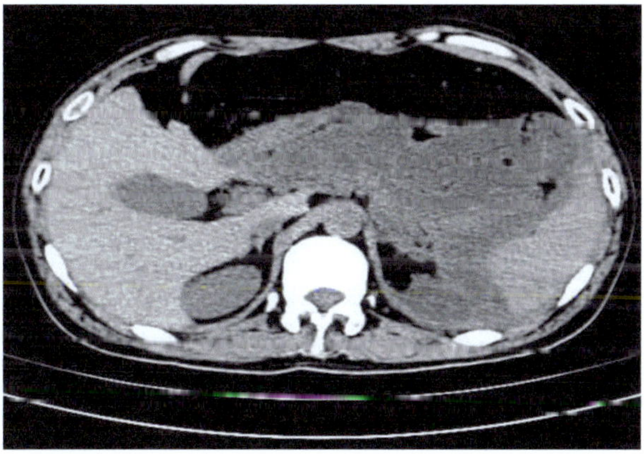

Fig. 6.5 The patient's preoperative CT revealed >50% pancreatic necrosis and a large amount of retroperitoneal effusion

in patients and combining the theories of damage control and pathway damage optimization, the author proposed the concept of drainage instead of removal and a posterior laparoscopic surgical approach.

Retroperitoneoscopic debridement and drainage of pancreatic necrotic tissue was performed in two phases. The left side was operated first, and the left side was operated using retroperitoneoscopic left adrenal surgery to establish the retroperitoneal space. Due to a large amount of fluid collection in the anterior pararenal space, the lateral cone fascia and perirenal fascia were perforated into the anterior pararenal space when blunt dissection of the abdominal wall muscles was performed using vascular forceps, a trocar of the abdominal wall was placed after sucking up a large amount of inflammatory fluid and necrotic tissue to establish pneumoperitoneum. The aspirator sucked up the effusion in the prerenal space, removed the pancreas and fat necrotic tissue as much as possible, and indwelled one double cannula and one latex drainage tube each for drainage (Fig. 6.6). Twenty-four days later, the patient underwent right surgery, and the right surgery was performed in the left lateral decubitus position. It first entered the retroperitoneal space to free the pararenal fat, free and enlarge the perirenal space. According to the preoperative image indicating the location of the effusion, the prerenal fascia was opened at the middle and lower pole of the kidney, entered the anterior pararenal space from the rear, the necrotic material and effusion in it were removed, and a double cannula was indwelled for drainage. Postoperative anti-inflammatory, enzyme suppression, and nutritional support treatment were given, and the patient was discharged with a significant reduction in postoperative pain and a smooth recovery (Fig. 6.7).

The retroperitoneal approach proposed by the author breaks through the limitations of conventional thinking, reaches the infected area through the route, avoids entering the abdominal cavity, reduces the spread of severe infection, does not excessively clean the necrotic tissue to reduce the additional damage to the normal tissue, and controls the damage within a certain range to reduce the systemic inflammatory response.

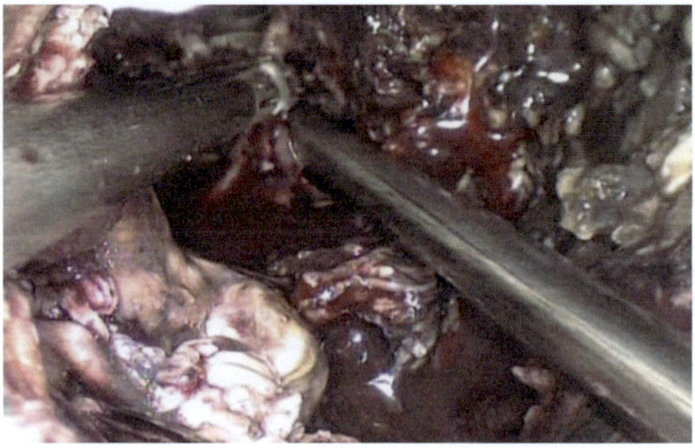

Fig. 6.6 Intraoperative removal of peripancreatic necrotic tissue

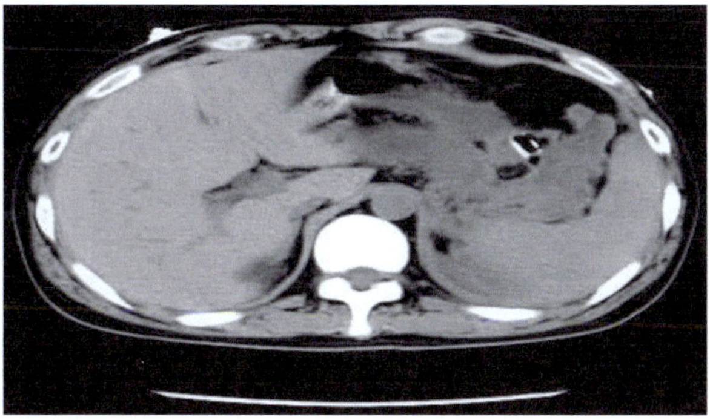

Fig. 6.7 Postoperative abdominal CT showed that the abdominal effusion was significantly eliminated

3 Resection Techniques

How to achieve complete, thorough and effective resection in resection surgery, especially radical surgery for malignant tumors, is a key aspect to ensure surgical results and improve patient prognosis. If the tumor does not achieve radical resection, residual tumor occurs, and tumor recurrence and metastasis are likely to occur after surgery, which greatly reduces the disease-free survival and overall survival of patients and is the main reason for the poor prognosis of patients. Among the resection techniques, the completeness and maneuverability of the resection are the two most concerned aspects for surgeons.

1. Completeness of resection

   The completeness of tumor resection includes the extent of lesion resection and the extent of lymph node dissection. In order to prevent the early recurrence and distant metastasis of pancreatic cancer and improve the prognosis of patients and improve the long-term survival rate of patients after radical surgery for pancreatic cancer, some scholars have proposed the concept of en bloc resection in pancreatic surgery, that is, en bloc resection of tissues including the pancreas and its surrounding lymph nodes and fat, to improve the R0 resection rate through complete resection specimens, so as to ensure the radical effect of surgery.

   By studying the characteristics of minimally invasive surgery, the author's team applied the concept of en bloc resection to minimally invasive radical surgery for pancreatic cancer by taking advantage of its magnified and flexible field of view and high level of refinement. (1) In pancreaticoduodenectomy lymph node dissection, the author often uses the common hepatic artery, proper hepatic artery, and portal vein as guidance and demarcation lines, first fully frees the lesser omental bursa tissue and groups 8a, 8p, and 12a lymph nodes near the left hepatoduodenal ligament and then turns them upwards to the left. The common hepatic artery, portal vein, and bile duct are suspended, respectively, and the perivascular adipose tissue and lymph nodes are completely removed. The above dissected lymph nodes and 12p lymph nodes are pulled together to the right posterior position of the portal vein for en bloc resection. When transecting the uncinate process of the pancreas, the nerve and lymph node tissues are tran-

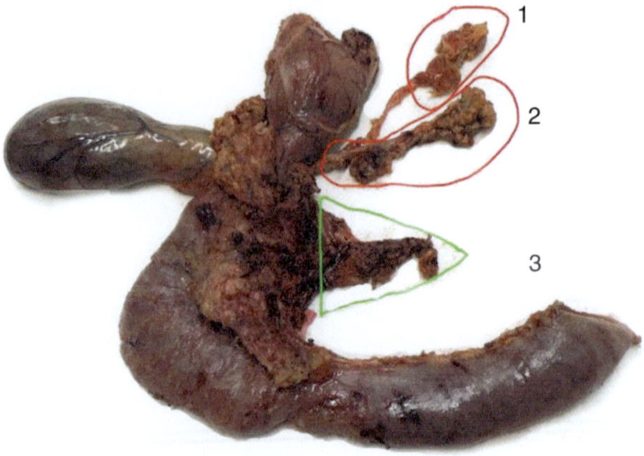

Fig. 6.8 En bloc pancreaticoduodenectomy. (*1*) Lesser peritoneal sac, 5 groups of lymph nodes; (*2*) 8a, 9, 12a lymph nodes; (*3*) 12p, 9, 14, 16 lymph nodes

sected from the cranial side of the foot abutting the right wall of the superior mesenteric artery, abdominal aorta, and celiac trunk using a bottom-up view angle of minimally invasive surgery, and the uncinate process is completely removed, and finally the specimen is removed en bloc together with the lymph nodes. The en bloc resection of pancreaticoduodenal specimens achieves en bloc and complete resection of lymph nodes while ensuring R0 resection, and gives full play to the advantages of minimally invasive surgery, which is safe and feasible to operate (Fig. 6.8). (2) Because of the lack of obvious symptoms, the malignant tumor of pancreatic body and tail is easy to infiltrate into retroperitoneal and surrounding organs. Moreover, the traditional operation of pancreatic body and tail does not completely remove the tissue between the posterior membrane of pancreas and renal fascia, which makes the resection rate of R0 low, and its therapeutic effect is often worse than that of pancreatic head tumor, and patients are prone to relapse after operation. Strasberg et al., at the University of Washington, USA, proposed radical antegrade modular pancreatosplenectomy (RAMPS) in 2003. RAMPS emphasizes the radical resection at peritoneal resection margin. According to whether the tumor invades the retropancreatic capsule, using the patterned anterior approach and posterior approach for resection range can effectively improve the R0 resection rate of retroperitoneal resection margin and radical effect of tumor. Compared with classic radical resection of pancreatic body and tail cancer, RAMPS shows greater improvement in R0 resection rate and 5-year survival rate of patients. Due to the wide range of RAMPS resections, which are demanding for the surgeon's anatomy and technique, they are rarely applied in minimally invasive surgery. The author's team applied RAMPS surgery in the field of laparoscopic and robotic minimally invasive surgery earlier, making full use of the advantages of laparoscopic and robotic facilities, through the intraoperative lens high-definition amplification effect and the fine operation of minimally invasive devices, in order to achieve a cleaner and complete resection, reduce the postoperative recurrence rate and prolong the survival time of patients. The author reported that after laparoscopic and robotic radical resection of pancreatic cancer, the R0 resection rate could reach 97.1% and

100%, the number of dissected lymph nodes was 10.5 and 11, respectively, and the overall survival time could reach 25 and 27 months after surgery.

2. Maneuverability of resection

   With the continuous development of instruments and minimally invasive techniques, the indications of minimally invasive surgery have been gradually extended to many fields of surgery and even can cover almost all surgical procedures. Due to different operating habits in different hospitals, there are great differences from the layout of Trocar hole to the selection of surgical approach, surgical instruments, and surgical steps, which is not conducive to the standardization of surgery, affects the promotion of surgery, and is not conducive to the unification of surgical quality and efficacy evaluation. The author's team summarized the experience of minimally invasive liver surgery, according to the different characteristics of liver surgery, developed the left lateral lobe, left liver, right liver, and other patterned surgical steps, to achieve the simplification and patterning of minimally invasive liver surgery. By summarizing and generalizing the surgical steps, and in order to further promote the use of patterned liver resection techniques in primary care units, the author's team has broken down the liver resection procedure into seven steps to perform: (1) the patient's position is placed in the supine position and operated according to the conventional four-hole method, and the specific body odor and trocar hole layout could be adjusted according to the specific circumstances of surgery; (2) the ligaments around the liver are sequentially divided to free the corresponding liver lobes to be removed; (3) the vascular pedicles entering the target liver segment or lobe are roughly separated and ligated or cut; (4) the liver tissue is cut and divided according to the selected liver; (5) the corresponding hepatic veins are roughly separated and divided; (6) the bleeding of the liver section is treated; (7) the drainage tube is indwelled to remove the resected liver specimens. By quantitatively describing the spatial relationship of blood vessels and bile ducts, the author performed "bundle" cutting and transection of the liver and hepatic duct together with the liver parenchyma to simplify laparoscopic left lateral lobectomy (Fig. 6.9),

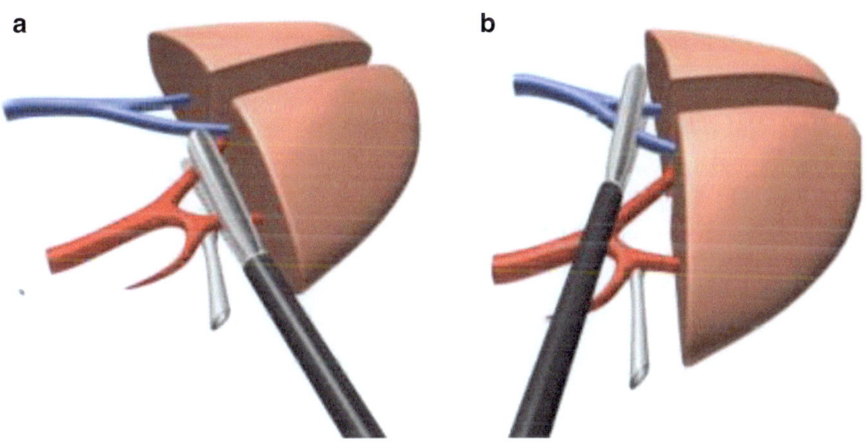

Fig. 6.9 Patterned left lateral lobectomy. (**a**) Transection into the hepatic blood flow; (**b**) Transection out of the hepatic blood flow

avoiding the high risk caused by anatomical porta hepatis, reducing the difficulty of surgery, simplifying the surgical mode, and popularizing laparoscopic left lateral lobectomy to county-level hospitals. For laparoscopic right hemihepatectomy with great difficulty in operation, the study data of the author team showed that the average operation time was 256.17 min, the average blood loss was 493.48 mL, and the average postoperative hospital stay was 8.91 days. Compared with open right hemihepatectomy, there was no serious complication. The operation time was not significantly increased compared with open surgery, but it significantly shortened the hospital stay, which was conducive to rapid recovery of patients after operation. Patterned hepatectomy technology simplifies and patterns complex laparoscopic hepatectomy, so that it can be more safe, effective, and convenient to be popularized to other primary medical institutions, which is helpful for the learning of the majority of medical colleagues.

3.1 Case 1

The patient, a 56-year-old man, was admitted to our hospital due to icteric skin and sclera for 15 days. Physical examination: temperature 36.8 °C, pulse rate 68 bpm, respiratory rate 18 bpm, blood pressure 140/85 mmHg. He's in a clear state of mind, acceptable nutritional status, and yellowing of the skin and sclera. The abdomen was slightly distended, the liver and spleen were not palpable under the ribs, no palpable mass, mild tenderness in the right upper quadrant, no rebound tenderness, normal bowel sounds, and negative shifting dullness. Blood biochemistry showed serum total bilirubin 325.3 μmol/L and direct bilirubin 264.8 μmol/L. CEA was 147.6 μg/L and CA19–9 was 285.3 KU/L. Preoperative contrast-enhanced MRI and PET-CT revealed a mass in the lower common bile duct, possible bile duct adenocarcinoma, and multiple retroperitoneal lymph node enlargement. The patient was clinically diagnosed with middle and lower bile duct cancer. Through the evaluation of the patient's general condition and systemic organ function, the patient had normal cardiopulmonary function and could tolerate surgical treatment. Through the analysis of imaging data, the patient's tumor was located in the lower bile duct and multiple retroperitoneal lymph nodes were enlarged. High-level evidence in evidence-based medicine recommended radical surgery. Combined with the experience and ability of the author's team in minimally invasive pancreaticoduodenectomy, various treatment methods, advantages, and disadvantages were explained to the patient and his family in detail, and the patient and his family chose to undergo robotic pancreaticoduodenectomy.

Surgical methods: After anesthesia, low leg lithotomy position was taken, pneumoperitoneum was established in the lower right part of the navel, and robotic surgical hole was patterned. In the operation, the gastrocolic ligament was first opened, a Kocher incision was performed, and the posterior aspect of the pancreatic head was fully mobilized until the celiac trunk and the right wall of the superior mesenteric artery. The vascular arch at the greater and lesser curvature of the stomach was divided, and the distal stomach was divided by a linear cutter stapler. According to the method of en bloc resection of lymph nodes, the lymph nodes near the hepatoduodenal ligament and celiac trunk were dissected, and the right gastric artery and gastroduodenal artery were properly divided. The gallbladder was mobilized retrogradely and the common bile duct was divided above the level of the cystic duct, and the upper resection margin of the bile duct was sent for frozen pathology, suggesting a negative resection margin. The gastrointestinal trunk vein was transected, the retropancreatic tunnel was opened, and the pancreas was transected with an ultrasonic scalpel. The initial segment of jejunum was freed, the mesojejunum was divided close to the intestinal wall at about 10 cm from the ligament of Treitz, the Kocher incision was continued, the dorsal and inferior sides of the pancreaticoduodenum were completely freed, the initial segment of jejunum was divided by a linear cutter stapler, and the initial segment of jejunum was pulled to the right from the inferior mesenteric hiatus. Attention was paid to protecting the superior mesenteric artery, the uncinate process and portal vein, common hepatic artery and paraceliac lymph nodes from below to above were completely removed, and en bloc resection of tumor specimens and lymph nodes was completed. Pancreaticojejunostomy, choledochojejunostomy, and gastrointestinal anastomosis were sequentially completed by the robot. The duration of surgery was 2.5 h, and the intraoperative blood loss was 100 mL. The patient recovered well postoperatively and was discharged on day 10. Pathological examination revealed adenocarcinoma of the lower bile duct with no tumor cells at the resection margin, and a total of 23 lymph nodes were dissected without metastatic lymph nodes. After follow-up, the patient has been 20 months since surgery, without tumor recurrence, and is in good physical condition.

Pancreaticoduodenectomy involves many organs and requires a large extent of resection. For the treatment of malignant tumors, ensuring negative resection margin and adequate extent of lymph node dissection is closely related to the prognosis of patients. Due to the special advantages of robotic surgery system compared with traditional laparoscopic surgery, the current surgery involving digestive tract reconstruction, including pancreaticoduodenectomy, has a significantly higher clinical recognition of robotic surgery than laparoscopic surgery. After accumulating a wealth of experience and skills in robotic surgery, the author compared the lymph node dissection between robotic and laparoscopic pancreaticoduodenectomy and concluded that the former has more advantages and is significantly superior to laparoscopic operation. This case also shows that minimally invasive en bloc resection technique can complete more thorough lymph node dissection and improve the R0 resection rate of the tumor, which is of great benefit to improve the disease-free survival and overall survival of patients and improve the prognosis of patients.

3.2 Case 2

The patient, a 42-year-old man, was admitted to our hospital due to bloating for half a year and examination revealed a tumor in the left lateral lobe of the liver for 7 days. Physical examination: temperature 36.5 °C, pulse rate 65 bpm, respiratory rate 16 bpm, blood pressure 130/80 mmHg. He was clearly conscious, cooperative on physical examination, with normal development, acceptable nutritional status, and no yellowing of the skin and sclera. The abdomen was flat, the liver and spleen were not palpable under the ribs, no palpable mass, no tenderness in the whole abdomen, no rebound tenderness, bowel sounds were normal, and shifting dullness was negative. The blood, urine, and stool routine were all normal. Blood biochemistry and tumor markers were normal. Contrast-enhanced MRI of the abdomen revealed a visible tumor in the left lateral lobe, approximately 8 × 8 cm, which was considered to be a hemangioma. The clinically diagnosis was hemangioma of the left lateral lobe of the liver. Through the evaluation of the patient's general condition and systemic organ function, the patient's cardiopulmonary function was normal, and the normal activity was not affected by the disease. Through the analysis of imaging data, the patient's tumor was located in the left lateral lobe of the liver, and the tumor compressed the stomach. At present, the patient has experienced bloating and other discomfort symptoms, with liver function of Child A, and can tolerate surgical treatment. The treatment methods as well as the advantages and disadvantages were explained to the patient and his family in detail, and the patient and his family chose to undergo laparoscopic left lateral lobectomy.

The author used patterned laparoscopic left lateral lobectomy to complete the operation. The patient was placed in the supine position, and after the completion of general anesthesia, pneumoperitoneum was established from the umbilicus, a 30° laparoscope was placed, and a four-hole method was taken for operation, with the main operation port located 10 cm below the left costal margin beside the rectus abdominis muscle. The right auxiliary operation hole was located 10 cm below the right costal margin beside the rectus abdominis muscle, and the left auxiliary operation hole was located near the anterior axillary line below the left costal margin. After exploration of the abdominal cavity, the ligamentum teres, falciform ligament, anterior lobe of the left coronary ligament, left deltoid ligament, posterior lobe of the left coronary ligament, and lesser omentum were sequentially divided using a harmonic scalpel until the root of the venous ligament, and the left lateral lobe of the liver was fully freed. The ultrasonic scalpel was used to dissect the anterior and upper and lower liver tissues of segment II/III vascular pedicle, and the thick separation of segment II/III vascular pedicle. II/III vascular pedicles were divided with a linear cutting sealer. Ultrasonic scalpel was used to dissect the upper and lower hepatic tissues of the left hepatic vein, and the left hepatic vein was separated coarsely. The left hepatic vein was transected using a linear vessel sealer. After adequate hemostasis of the liver wound, no drainage tube was left in place. The hemangioma specimen was crushed and removed from the enlarged umbilical incision. The patient recovered uneventfully after surgery and was discharged from the hospital 2 days after surgery.

The difference between patterned left lateral lobectomy and other procedures is that a coarse separation of the hepatic entry and exit vessels is proposed, rather than a fine separation of the intrahepatic ducts, followed by division of the surrounding liver tissue together. By simplifying and modeling the procedure, we are able to minimize the chance of intraoperative vascular injury, significantly reduce the difficulty of the procedure, shorten the learning curve of the surgeons, and make the quality of the procedure more uniform and suitable for implementation in primary units.

4 Reconstruction Techniques

Surgical procedures usually also require the use of reconstruction techniques, including digestive tract reconstruction, vascular reconstruction, urethral reconstruction, and so on. Reconstruction surgery is a key step to restore the patency of the tube and ensure organ function. The quality of reconstruction is closely related to the postoperative anastomotic healing, complications, and prognosis of patients. Good anastomosis technique is not only beneficial to accelerate the healing of each anastomosis, promote the recovery of organ function, reduce the incidence of postoperative complications, but also simplify the operation steps and shorten the operation time.

Pancreaticoduodenectomy is known as the operation with the most steps and the highest difficulty in abdominal surgery due to its involvement in the reconstruction of three anastomoses: pancreatico (pancreaticogastric), biliary-enteric, and gastrointestinal anastomoses. Because the poor healing of each anastomotic stoma will lead to corresponding postoperative complications, such as: pancreatic leakage, bile leakage, gastrointestinal anastomotic leakage, etc., these complications on the one hand prolong the hospital stay of patients and increase the hospital costs of patients; on the other hand, anastomotic leakage is easy to corrode the corresponding surrounding blood vessels and tissues, which may cause more serious complications such as postoperative bleeding or infection, and even threaten the lives of patients. Among them, pancreatic leakage is the main cause of poor prognosis, and pancreaticojejunostomy reconstruction is also a challenging way of digestive tract reconstruction, which seriously hinders the development and promotion of pancreaticoduodenectomy. Surgeons have made a variety of attempts in the reconstruction of pancreaticojejunostomy, resulting in a variety of novel anastomosis methods, however so far there is no anastomosis method that can completely avoid pancreatic leakage. Combined with the reconstruction experience in open and minimally invasive pancreaticoduodenectomy, the author's team changed the previous traditional concept of pursuing strict mechanical suture, from the perspective of protecting the anastomosis, reducing the tension of the anastomosis, and reducing the penetrating injury to the pancreas, through conceptual innovation and repeated optimization in practice, from the initial 1 + 2 pancreaticojejunostomy, a single needle full-thickness pancreatic anastomosis method was formed. The core technology of this new anastomosis method is to use U-shaped suture of pancreatic stump to reduce the extravasation of pancreatic branch pancreatic duct on the pancreatic section; 1 needle 4-0 prolene suture is used to continuously suture the whole layer of pancreatic stump and the serous layer of jejunum; the pancreatic duct and jejunal mucosa are aligned to replace the anastomosis mode of mucosa to mucosa (Fig. 6.10). This method is simple and feasible under minimally invasive conditions

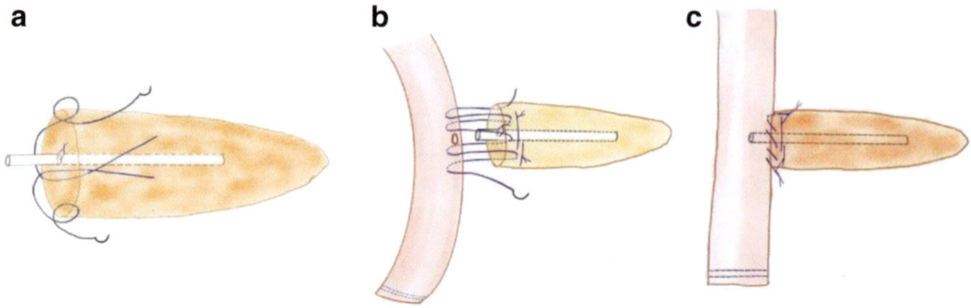

Fig. 6.10 Single-layer pancreatojejunostomy. (**a**) Two figure-eight sutures traversed the pancreas in full thickness. (**b**) A single layer of the continuous suture between the pancreatic stump and the jejunum was performed. (**c**) Anterior view of the pancreaticojejunal anastomosis

and suitable for minimally invasive surgery. The incidence of postoperative pancreatic leakage is low, with good safety and effectiveness. According to the clinical study data of the author's team, the incidence of clinically relevant pancreatic fistula after robotic pancreaticoduodenectomy using 1 + 2 pancreaticojejunostomy was 9.35%, while no clinically relevant pancreatic fistula occurred after single-needle full-thickness pancreatic anastomosis, which was significantly lower than the incidence of clinically relevant pancreatic leakage after laparotomy (16.3%), laparoscopy (12.1%), and robotics (11%) reported in the previous literature.

In the traditional surgical concept, when the pancreatic duct of the pancreas is damaged, pancreaticojejunostomy, salvage distal pancreatectomy, and even pancreaticoduodenectomy are required because the pancreatic duct cannot heal spontaneously, so that the operation loses more normal pancreatic tissue and may have a greater impact on its own pancreatic function after surgery. In order to reduce surgical trauma and protect the function of the pancreas, the author's team took the lead in implementing main pancreatic duct bridge repair, avoiding the large traumatic loss of the pancreas due to pancreatectomy. On the basis of successful operation, the author established the innovative bridge closure theory in pancreatic anastomosis by referring to the bridge construction process in the engineering building, and pancreatic end-to-end anastomosis reconstruction can be performed for middle pancreatectomy. Through this technique, the normal pancreatic tissue can be preserved to the greatest extent, the integrity of pancreatic physiological function and anatomical structure can be ensured, which is conducive to the long-term prognosis of patients. The anastomosis theory is expected to change the traditional treatment of benign pancreatic diseases.

4.1 Case 1

The patient, a 37-year-old man, was admitted to our hospital due to icteric skin and sclera for 20 days. Physical examination: temperature 36.5 °C, pulse rate 76 bpm, respiratory rate 16 bpm, blood pressure 128/80 mmHg. He was clearly conscious, acceptable nutritional status, and yellowing of the skin and sclera. The abdomen was flat, the liver and spleen were not palpable under the ribs, no palpable mass, mild tenderness in the right upper quadrant, no rebound tenderness, bowel sounds were normal, and shifting dullness was negative. Blood biochemistry showed serum total bilirubin 343.3 μmol/L and direct bilirubin 284.2 μmol/L. CA19–9 was 196.7 KU/L. Preoperative contrast-enhanced MRI revealed a mass in the lower common bile duct and the possibility of bile duct adenocarcinoma, which was clinically suspected to be middle and lower bile duct cancer. Through the assessment of the patient's general condition and systemic organ function, the patient was able to tolerate surgical treatment. Through the analysis of imaging data, the patient's tumor was located in the lower bile duct. Through the preoperative comprehensive evaluation of the patient's disease risk, surgical risk, treatment timing, treatment plan, the experience and ability of the surgical team, as well as the mastery of the intervention means, various treatment methods and advantages and disadvantages were explained to the patient and his family in detail, and the patient and his family chose to undergo robotic pancreaticoduodenectomy.

Surgical methods: After completing the patterning for robotic surgery, the gastrocolic ligament was first opened and a Kocher incision was made to fully free the posterior aspect of the pancreatic head until the abdominal trunk and the right wall of the superior mesenteric artery. The vascular arch at the greater and lesser curvature of the stomach was divided, and the distal stomach was divided by a linear cutter stapler. According to the method of en bloc resection of lymph nodes, lymph nodes near the hepatoduodenal ligament and celiac axis were dissected. The gallbladder was retrogradely mobilized, the common bile duct was transected above the level of the cystic duct, and the tumor was found to invade the portal vein wall up to 2 cm when the extrahepatic bile duct was freed, requiring portal vein resection and reconstruction to complete radical surgery. The posterior pancreatic tunnel was opened and the pancreas was transected with an ultrasonic scalpel. The initial segment of the jejunum was divided approximately 10 cm from the ligament of Treitz, and the initial segment of the jejunum was pulled to the right from the inferior mesenteric hiatus. The right wall of the superior mesenteric artery was abutted, and the uncinate process was completely removed from bottom to top. The upper and lower ends of the invaded portal vein were clamped with vascular forceps, and about 3 cm of the portal vein was removed. Intraoperative frozen upper and lower resection margins revealed negative resection margins, and en bloc resection of the pancreaticoduodenum, invaded portal vein, and lymph nodes was completed. In the reconstruction stage, continuous portal vein end-to-end anastomosis was first performed using a 5-0 Prolene suture, and the portal vein was opened after the completion of vascular suture, with smooth blood flow and no exudation. The posterior wall of the pancreaticojejunum was continuously sutured with 4-0 Prolene suture, and after the pancreatic duct was built and reinforced with two stitches superiorly and inferiorly, the anterior wall of the pancreaticojejunum was continued to be continuously sutured to complete the 1 + 2 pancreaticojejunostomy. 5-0 Prolene suture was used for continuous single-layer suture in biliary-enteric anastomosis, and 4-0 Prolene suture was used for continuous suture to close the opening site after gastrointestinal anastomosis with cutter stapler. The whole operation duration was 6 h, and the intraoperative blood loss was 200 mL. Postoperative abdominal ultrasonography revealed patent blood flow. The patient had smooth food intake and extubation after operation and was discharged 10 days after surgery. There was no bleeding or second admission after discharge.

In this case of pancreaticoduodenectomy with combined resection and reconstruction, because the tumor invades the portal vein, it is not only necessary to complete the en bloc resection of the tumor specimen and portal vein wall, but also to complete the reconstruction of the portal vein, pancreaticojejunum, biliary-enteric, and gastrointestinal anastomosis during the operation. The requirements for the reconstruction technique are rarely reported internationally. The author deeply analyzed the anatomical characteristics and healing principle of different anastomotic tissues and successfully completed this operation after accumulating a large number of robotic surgical experience and reconstruction skills, confirming the safety and feasibility of this surgical method and technique. In the long-term surgical practice, the author also completed the simplification of reconstruction technique for different anastomoses, which is convenient for the implementation and promotion of the technique.

4.2 Case 2

A 55-year-old female patient was admitted due to space-occupying lesions in the neck of pancreas found by physical examination for 10 days. Physical examination: temperature 36.9 °C, pulse rate 63 bpm, respiratory rate 17 bpm, blood pressure 145/95 mmHg. The patient had clear consciousness and good nutritional status. The abdomen was distended, the liver and spleen were not palpable under the ribs, no palpable mass, no tenderness in the whole abdomen, no rebound tenderness, normal bowel sounds, and negative shifting dullness. Blood, urine and stool routine, blood biochemistry, and tumor markers were normal. PET-CT examination revealed slightly hypodense nodules in the neck of the pancreas, considering benign or low-grade malignant lesions. Contrast-enhanced magnetic resonance imaging of the pancreas revealed a small nodule of about 11 mm × 9 mm at the junction of the head and neck of the pancreas, which was considered to be a low-grade malignant tumor, with the greatest possibility of neuroendocrine tumors and no abnormal stenosis or dilatation of the pancreatic duct. Based on the patient's preoperative imaging findings, a clinical diagnosis of pancreatic neuroendocrine tumor was suspected. Various treatment modalities and advantages and disadvantages were explained to the patient and her family in detail, and the patient and her family chose to undergo robotic mid-pancreatectomy.

Surgical methods: The operation was performed in the head high foot low lithotomy position. After completing the pneumoperitoneum and Trocar layout, the abdominal and pelvic organs were explored without metastasis or abnormality. The gastrocolic ligament was incised to fully expose each segment of the pancreas, and intraoperative ultrasound was applied to confirm that the tumor was located in the neck of the pancreas. The superior and inferior margins of the pancreas were separated 1 cm from the right side of the tumor, the superior mesenteric vein and splenic vein were exposed and protected, and the tunnel behind the pancreas was freed. 1 cm away from the left and right sides of the tumor, the middle pancreas and main pancreatic duct were transected with an ultrasonic scalpel. After cauterization and hemostasis of the broken end of the pancreas, the examination of the wound showed that the pancreatic juice overflowed from the broken end of the distal pancreatic duct, with a distance of about 3.5 cm from the broken end on both sides. A plastic support tube of the pancreatic duct with a length of about 10 cm and a diameter of 1.2 mm was selected and placed in the pancreatic ducts on both sides, and the broken ends of the pancreas on both sides were fully freed to ensure that there was no tension on the broken ends of the coapted pancreas. 5-0 Porlene suture was used to suture the broken ends of pancreatic ducts on both sides, and 4-0 Prolene suture was used to continuously suture the broken ends of pancreas on both sides. It was confirmed that there was no significant bleeding or pancreatic fistula at the anastomosis, and a drainage tube was placed in the surgical area for drainage. The operation time was 105 min, and the intraoperative bleeding was about 50 mL. Postoperative symptomatic treatments such as fasting, anti-inflammatory, acid suppression, enzyme suppression, and nutritional support were given. The patient had only a small amount of biochemical leakage after surgery, without clinically relevant pancreatic leakage or other postoperative complications, and was discharged on the seventh postoperative day after good recovery.

The pancreas not only has a deep anatomical location and is surrounded by abundant adjacent blood vessels, but also has endocrine and exocrine functions. Therefore, surgical treatment of pancreatic tumors should not only consider the radicality of tumor resection, but also pay attention to protecting normal pancreatic function. For benign or low-grade malignant tumors of the neck and body of the pancreas, mid-pancreatectomy is required to avoid adverse effects on the quality of life and long-term prognosis of patients after surgery. Traditional middle-segment pancreatectomy requires the completion of anastomosis between the distal pancreas and the digestive tract; however, the incidence of anastomotic complications between the pancreas and the digestive tract is high, and the physiological structure of the normal pancreas is changed. Compared with the traditional reconstruction method, the author avoided the direct contact between pancreatic juice and gastrointestinal juice and reduced the probability of complications such as bleeding and pancreatic leakage to a certain extent. Through the placement of pancreatic duct support tube, the process of end-to-end anastomosis of pancreatic duct is more convenient, which is conducive to the drainage of pancreatic juice and the prevention of postoperative pancreatic duct stenosis, and can effectively promote the recovery of patients and improve the prognosis.

Suggested Reading

Chen P, Tang C. Treatment of severe acute pancreatitis by laparoscopic posterior drainage. Chin J Curr Adv Gen Surg. 2009;12(11):928–30.

Chen YJ, Lai EC, Lau WY, et al. Enteric reconstruction of pancreatic stump following pancreaticoduodenectomy: a review of the literature. Int J Surg. 2014;12(7):706–11.

Ecker BL, McMillan MT, Asbun HJ, et al. Characterization and optimal management of high-risk pancreatic anastomoses during pancreatoduodenectomy. Ann Surg. 2018;267(4):608–16.
Liu R. Laparoscopic regular hepatectomy. J Surg Concepts Pract. 2004;6:450–2.
Liu R. Development and current status of total laparoscopic hepatectomy in mainland China: a multicenter 14-year experience. Chin J Laparosc Surg. 2009;2(1):5–13.
Liu R. Reasonable selection and evaluation of laparoscopic hepatectomy approach. Chin J Laparosc Surg. 2018a;11(3):129–31.
Liu R. Experience and lessons of 1010 cases of robotic pancreatic surgery. J South Med Univ. 2018b;2(38).
Liu R, Hu MG. Technical points of laparoscopic right hemihepatectomy. Chin J Pract Surg. 2010;30(8):654–6.
Liu R, Liu Q. Intraoperative risk and prognostic control and minimally invasive hepatopancreatobiliary surgery. Chin J Laparosc Surg. 2017;10(2):65–7.
Liu R, Zhao GD. The "gold standard" procedure for left hepatic lobectomy: laparoscopic left hepatic lobectomy. Chin J Laparosc Surg. 2010;3(6):474–8.
Liu R, Zhao GD. Liver anatomy: from the trunk theory under static anatomy of cadavers to the watershed theory under morphology of clinical potential. Chin J Laparosc Surg. 2018;11(5):257–60.
Liu R, Wang YH, Zhou NX, et al. Laparoscopic left hepatectomy: a case report. Chin J Pract Surg. 2002;10:61.
Liu R, Wang YH, Zhou NX, et al. Total laparoscopic anatomical left hemihepatectomy: a report of 3 cases. Chin J Pract Surg. 2003;(9):47–8.
Liu R, Hu MG, Wang G. Total laparoscopic right tri-lobectomy: a case report. Natl Med J China. 2005;25:1783.
Liu R, Xu DB, Luo Y, et al. Laparoscopic excision of lesser omental cyst: a case report. Natl Med J China. 2007;48:3456.
Liu R, Zhao GD, Ma X, Hu MG, Wang W. Application of retroperitoneoscopic technique in surgical treatment of severe acute pancreatitis. Chin J Laparosc Surg. 2010;3(4):309–12.
Liu R, Zhang X, Zhao GD, et al. Retroperitoneoscopic pancreatic surgery: from imagination to clinical application. Chin J Laparosc Surg. 2011;04(6):426–30.
Liu R, Zhao GD, Yin ZZ, et al. Case report of robotic pancreatic tumor enucleation combined with main pancreatic duct bridge repair. Chin J Laparosc Surg. 2016a;9(06):373–4.
Liu R, Song YY, Zhao GD, et al. A case report of robotic pancreaticoduodenectomy combined with portal vein resection and reconstruction. Chin J Laparosc Surg. 2016b;9(2):124–5.
Liu R, Yin ZZ, Zhao GD, et al. Laparoscopic or robotic resection of pancreatic caudal tumor via splenocolic ligament approach. J Laparosc Surg. 2017a;22(01):66–9.
Liu R, Zhao GD, Yin ZZ. Theory and skills of robotic LR type 1 + 2 pancreaticojejunostomy: a report of 104 cases. Chin J Surg. 2017b;10(01):7–10.
Liu R, Zhang T, Zhao ZM, et al. The surgical outcomes of robot-assisted laparoscopic pancreaticoduodenectomy versus laparoscopic pancreaticoduodenectomy for periampullary neoplasms: a comparative study of a single center. Surg Endosc. 2017c;31(6):2380–6.
Liu R, Liu Q, Zhao ZM, et al. Robotic versus laparoscopic distal pancreatectomy: a propensity score-matched study. J Surg Oncol. 2017d;116(4):461–9.
Liu R, Wang ZZ, Gao YX, et al. A case report of "Rong" robotic mid-pancreatectomy. Chin J Laparosc Surg. 2017e;10(5):319–20.
Liu R, Liu Q, Zhao ZM, et al. Application of single-needle full-layer pancreaticojejunostomy (301 type) in pancreaticoduodenectomy. J Laparosc Surg. 2018a;23(11):854–7.
Liu R, Wang ZZ, Gao YX, et al. Application of end-to-end anastomosis in robotic central pancreatectomy. J Vis Exp. 2018b;(136):57495.
Liu Q, Zhao ZM, Gao YX, Zhao GD, Tan XL, Liu R. Novel single-layer continuous suture of Pancreaticojejunostomy for robotic pancreaticoduodenectomy. J Hepatobiliary Pancreat Sci. 2020;27(2):56–63.
Liu Q, Zhao ZM, Gao YX, Zhao GD, Jiang N, Lau WY, Liu R. A novel technique for single layer pancreatojejunostomy is not inferior to modified Blumgart anastomosis in robotic pancreatoduodenectomy results of a randomized controlled trial. Ann Surg Oncol. 2021;28(4):2346–55.

Pedrazzoli SJM. Pancreatoduodenectomy (PD) and postoperative pancreatic fistula (POPF): a systematic review and analysis of the POPF-related mortality rate in 60,739 patients retrieved from the English literature published between 1990 and 2015. Medicine (Baltimore). 2017;96(19):e6858.
Qu L, Zhiming Z, Xianglong T, et al. Short- and mid-term outcomes of robotic versus laparoscopic distal pancreatosplenectomy for pancreatic ductal adenocarcinoma: a retrospective propensity score-matched study. Int J Surg. 2018;55:81–6.
Rong L. Establishment of surgical method and optimization of technique for LR-type robotic pancreaticoduodenectomy. Chin J Laparosc Surg. 2016a;4(9):193–5.
Rong L. Establishment of surgical method and optimization of technique for LR-type robotic pancreaticoduodenectomy. Chin J Laparosc Surg. 2016b;9(4):193–5.
Shin SH, Kim YJ, Song KB, et al. Totally laparoscopic or robot-assisted pancreaticoduodenectomy versus open surgery for periampullary neoplasms: separate systematic reviews and meta-analyses. Surg Endosc. 2017;31(9):3459–74.
Strasberg SM, Drebin JA, Linehan D. Radical antegrade modular pancreatosplenectomy. Surgery. 2003;133(5):521–7.
Strasberg SM, Linehan DC, Hawkins WG. Radical antegrade modular pancreatosplenectomy procedure for adenocarcinoma of the body and tail of the pancreas: ability to obtain negative tangential margins. J Am Coll Surg. 2007;204(2):244–9.
Sun B, Cheng ZX, Jia G. New highlights in the treatment of severe acute pancreatitis: multidisciplinary and minimally invasive. Chin J Pract Surg. 2012;32(7):525–7.
Wang G, Liu R. Clinical comparative study of laparoscopic and open hepatectomy. Chin J Pract Surg. 2005;10:617–20.
Wang YH, Liu R, Zhou NX, et al. Anatomical basis and technical problems of total laparoscopic regular hepatectomy. Chin J Gen Surg. 2003;7:17–9.
Wang XF, Hu MG, Zhao GD, et al. Exploration of a laparoscopic standard: patterned laparoscopic left hemihepatectomy. Chin J Endosc Surg. 2014;3:160–6.
Wang X, Hu M, Zhao Z, et al. An improved surgical technique for pure laparoscopic left hemihepatectomy: ten years experience in a tertiary center. J Laparoendosc Adv Surg Tech A. 2016;26(11):862–9.
Xu Y, Hu MG, Zhao GD, et al. Patterned laparoscopic right hemihepatectomy. Chin J Endosc Surg. 2015;8(4):237–41.
Xu D, Jiang KR, Lu ZP, et al. Clinical efficacy of radical antegrade modular pancreatosplenectomy in the treatment of pancreatic body and tail cancer. Chin J Digest Surg. 2016;15(6):567–73.
Zhang T, Zhao ZM, Gao YX, et al. The learning curve for a surgeon in robot-assisted laparoscopic pancreaticoduodenectomy: a retrospective study in a high-volume pancreatic center. Surg Endosc. 2019;33(9):2927–33.
Zhao GD, Hu MG, Liu R. Patterned laparoscopic left lateral lobectomy: a report of 71 cases. J South Med Univ. 2011;4:737–40.
Zhao GD, Liu R, Ma X, et al. Retroperitoneal laparoscopic pancreatectomy: a report of 4 cases. Chin J Pract Surg. 2012a;01:85–7.
Zhao G, Xue R, Ma X, et al. Retroperitoneoscopic pancreatectomy: a new surgical option for pancreatic disease. Surg Endosc. 2012b;26(6):1609–16.
Zhao G, Hu M, Liu R, et al. Two anatomical pathways for retroperitoneoscopic pancreatectomy: indications for the posterior and lateral approaches. World J Surg. 2014a;38(11):3023–32.
Zhao G, Hu M, Liu R, et al. Single-port retroperitoneoscopic pancreatectomy: preliminary results from the first 3 patients. J Clin Gastroenterol. 2014b;48(6):559–62.
Zhao G, Hu M, Liu R, et al. Retroperitoneoscopic anatomical necrosectomy: a modified single-stage video-assisted retroperitoneal approach for treatment of infected necrotizing pancreatitis. Surg Innov. 2015;22(4):360–5.
Zhao G, Wang Z, Hu M, et al. Preliminary clinical experience with robotic retroperitoneoscopic pancreatic surgery. World J Surg Oncol. 2018;16(1):171.

MIX
Papier aus verantwortungsvollen Quellen
Paper from responsible sources
FSC® C105338

If you have any concerns about our products,
you can contact us on
ProductSafety@springernature.com

In case Publisher is established outside the EU,
the EU authorized representative is:
Springer Nature Customer Service Center GmbH
Europaplatz 3, 69115 Heidelberg, Germany

Printed by Libri Plureos GmbH
in Hamburg, Germany